The
Ovulation
Method
of Birth Regulation

The Ovulation Method of Birth Regulation

The Latest Advances for Achieving or Postponing Pregnancy—Naturally

MERCEDES ARZÚ WILSON

VNR VAN NOSTRAND REINHOLD COMPANY

NEW YORK   CINCINNATI   ATLANTA   DALLAS   SAN FRANCISCO

LONDON   TORONTO   MELBOURNE

While every effort has been made to provide dependable information, the publisher and author cannot be held responsible for any errors or omissions.

Van Nostrand Reinhold Company Regional Offices:
New York   Cincinnati   Atlanta   Dallas   San Francisco

Van Nostrand Reinhold Company International Offices:
London   Toronto   Melbourne

Copyright © 1980 by Litton Educational Publishing, Inc.

Library of Congress Catalog Card Number: 79-15167
ISBN : 0-442-29515-4

Manufactured in the United States of America

Published by Van Nostrand Reinhold Company
135 West 50th Street, New York, N.Y. 10020

Published simultaneously in Canada by Van Nostrand Reinhold Ltd.

15 14 13 12 11 10 9 8 7 6 5 4 3 2 1

Library of Congress Cataloging in Publication Data

Wilson, Mercedes Arzú.
    The ovulation method of birth regulation.

    Includes index.
    1. Rhythm method (Birth control) 2. Ovulation—Detection.
    3. Cervix mucus. 4. Menstrual cycle.
I. Title. [DNLM: 1. Rhythm methods. WP630 W75lo]
RG136.5.W54   613.9′434   79-15167
ISBN 0-442-29515-4

To all the members of my family who gave me their untiring support and encouragement, and to all the scientists and teachers who have voluntarily given their time and effort to perfect this method and to spread this knowledge to every woman in the world.

Foreword

Lyn and I are pleased to place on record the deep affection, respect and gratitude we feel towards Mercedes Wilson, and to acknowledge her special place in the history of the development of the Ovulation Method. When she was first introduced to it she felt that this knowledge should be in the possession of all adolescent and mature women, so that they need no longer regard their reproductive physiology as incomprehensible or frightening. She was able also to see that the Ovulation Method could be of inestimable help in the solution of problems of fertility regulation in the developing countries—she was thinking of her native Guatemala particularly—and she devised a recording method which we immediately adopted because it provides an international language by which even totally illiterate women can record their cervical mucus observations. Additional impetus was given to her work by the widespread recognition of the multiple harmful effects which have followed the implementation of programs of contraception and abortion, and of the fact that the programs were often implemented without proper concern for the dignity and freedom of the individuals concerned. Sooner or later it will be acknowledged that the only truly successful solution to these problems will be found in the use of a natural method, the knowledge being provided by a competent teacher who both accepts, and defends, the right of the husband and wife to use or not to use it, according to their own estimates of their needs.

It is a biological fact that a woman is incapable of conceiving most of the time. In a fertile cycle she has a fertile phase of one or perhaps several days. If there is no intimate sexual contact with a male during this fertile phase she will not conceive—that fact is self-evident. Some people have been reluctant to accept sexual discipline, but gradually it has come to be understood that self-control is necessary to the achievement of psychological maturity, and that at the heart of loving is generosity towards the beloved person. Natural family planning fosters communication and cooperation between the husband and wife, and thereby promotes the development of those virtues which are essential to the stability and happiness of marriage. If family life is secure and adult people have learned to be unselfish and thoughtful, the whole of society will benefit—there will gradually occur the relief of poverty, care of the oppressed and handicapped and old people, the correction of injustice, and perhaps peace will come at last.

The Ovulation Method is the most modern of the natural methods of family planning, and one which has been the subject of thorough scientific research. It remains for it to be taught correctly by teachers who are motivated to its success, so that they will teach with care, confidence and that encouragement which is engendered by deep concern for the true welfare of those who seek their assistance. The method is effective if the teachers meet these requirements and the husbands and wives are prepared to make an effort to succeed.

I hope that this book will be widely read. It is the story not only of the Ovulation Method itself, but of a very remarkable woman who has shown extraordinary fortitude and endurance in her efforts to assist the under-privileged. Her zeal is that of a person who stamps society with her own mark, who sees and answers a need; like all those people who have effected lasting good in human affairs she has remained constant in the face of jealousy and uninformed criticism. The book is also a tribute to those wonderful people who have responded to her inspiring leadership and who will help her continue her work far into the future.

J. J. BILLINGS, PRESIDENT, WOOMB INTERNATIONAL

Dr. John Billings, K.C.S.G., Head, Department of Neurology, St. Vincent's Hospital, Melbourne, Australia; Physician in Charge, Medical Clinic, Royal Victorian Eye and Ear Hospital; Former Chairman, Medical Research Advisory Committee, National Health and Medical Health Research Council, Melbourne, Australia; Senior Consultant, Natural Family Planning Clinic, St. Vincent's Hospital, Melbourne, Australia; Dean, Clinical School, St. Vincent's Hospital, University of Melbourne, Faculty of Medicine.

Preface

From 1968 to 1970, because of my husband's involvement in oil exploration, my family and I lived in Melbourne, Australia. It was there, in 1969, that I first heard of the Ovulation Method of natural family planning—from a small news item in the back pages of the Melbourne paper, *The Age.* The item described a new natural method of birth control, developed by a Melbourne husband-and-wife team, Dr. John Billings and Dr. Evelyn Billings, and told of classes that were held on the subject. My husband and I attended one of the classes, and what we learned there revolutionized our thinking and our way of life.

At the 45-minute lecture, Dr. Evelyn Billings outlined the Ovulation Method, explaining that it is based on the fact that during the days a woman is capable of conceiving, she always has a particular mucous secretion from the glands of the neck of the uterus that she is able to recognize. Since the mucous secretion heralds the approach of ovulation, through their decision either to have intercourse or to abstain from it during the fertile period, a couple is able to achieve or to postpone pregnancy without having to use oral or mechanical contraceptive devices of any kind.

In the weeks following that meeting, my interest in the method grew, both for personal reasons and because I saw that the method would be of great value to people in my native country, Guatemala, and in other developing countries as well.

At the end of 1970, while awaiting our resident visa for the United States where my husband had been transferred, we spent a few months in Guatemala, where I started teaching the Ovulation Method to my friends and relatives. I also gave a formal presentation of the method at a meeting of the Christian Family Movement in Guatemala City. It was the largest meeting ever of the organization, a fact that made me aware of the great interest people had in natural methods of family planning.

Soon after, I was asked to teach in various parts of Guatemala. I agreed to do so, deciding to concentrate on the poorer parishes on the outskirts of Guatemala City. In the beginning, I was mainly interested in promulgating the Ovulation Method to the poor, but later, I became interested in disseminating information about the Ovulation Method to everyone I could reach.

The response to the lectures I gave was enthusiastic. One of my most vivid memories is that of a parish priest who stripped the altar to turn his church into a lecture room. He had gathered together about 100 people, mostly women, some children, a few men. We lectured to these people as a group and then divided them into small groups to make it easier for them to ask questions more privately. We were happy to find out, from the questions and comments, that the people easily understood the method.

From experience gathered in that and other lectures, effective methods of teaching people of little education and sophistication were devised. I developed a simple method of charting data about the menstrual cycle (see page 37) that could be used by people unable to read or write, a group that makes up a large percentage of the world population.

In 1970 it was arranged that the Billingses would lecture in Guatemala to the general public, and also attempt to make doctors aware of this new method of family planning. The Billingses lectured extensively throughout Guatemala, in other Central American countries, and in Mexico. The interest in these lectures was remarkable. People came in hundreds—and sometimes in thousands—to hear them.

After their Central American tour, the Billingses came to Washington, at the invitation of Aid for International Development and the Human Life Foundation, to meet in person and by telephone conference with various members of the scientific community who were interested in promulgating various methods of birth control. Thus the Ovulation Method came to the attention of a wider scientific community. During this visit to the United States, the Billingses also lectured to a medical group in Los Angeles sponsored by the Archdiocese. In 1972, they again lectured in the United States, and in 1973 they returned to Washington to attend a conference sponsored by the Human Life Foundation.

In 1971 my family and I moved to Covington, Louisiana, a suburb of New Orleans, where we now live. Soon after settling in, I resumed my work with the Ovulation Method, giving bimonthly lectures and quarterly workshops to train teachers. In addition to people from Louisiana, the audiences included couples, individual women, and doctors from other states who returned to their towns and cities to teach and train others. Soon requests for me to lecture poured in from all parts of the United States, Canada, and Latin America. To make the most of my time, I finally was forced to confine my work to teacher-training courses rather than to lectures, which aroused interest but made no provision for follow-up.

On January 27, 1977, the World Organization of the Ovulation Method—Billings (WOOMB) was inaugurated at a meeting in Los Angeles by a group of teachers of the Ovulation Method from Australia, Canada, the United States, Latin America, and the Far East. The main objective of WOOMB was set forth as the dissemination of accurate information about the Ovulation Method to every woman of child-bearing age throughout the world.

In June, 1977, the United States branch of the organization was established. The United States branch was divided into regions, and it was planned that quarterly teacher-training workshops would be held in each region and that workshops would be well advertised in newspapers and other media.

At this writing, the Ovulation Method has spread to 100 countries around the world and there are several hundred trained teachers of the Ovulation Method in the United States. The number of women who have been taught the Ovulation Method is undetermined at the moment, but there are plans underway to gather and evaluate statistics from all over the United States. (L.A. study "Time Magazine.")

The organization of WOOMB into an international body with a U.S. branch has enabled promoters of the Ovulation Method to present their philosophy and goals accurately, and it has encouraged uniformity of teaching. With national and international representation, WOOMB hopes to qualify for funds from the U.S. government and international organizations that would help provide the volunteer teachers with the literature, and audiovisual equipment needed to teach the method efficiently.

Such is the present state of the Ovulation Method. It is my fervent hope that this book will spread the good news of a natural, simple, safe and effective method of family planning that can be used by all women.

Mercedes Arzú Wilson, President, WOOMB
Covington, Louisiana

Introduction

The Ovulation Method was developed because of a pressing need to improve on the Rhythm (Calendar) and Temperature methods of Natural Family Planning. Dr. John Billings and Father Maurice Catarinich, working in Melbourne during the 1950s, had extensively appraised these two earlier methods with particular emphasis on the thorough investigation of unplanned pregnancies. This appraisal included the testing of all possible modifications and combinations of the two methods and the formulation of optimum rules for their application. These workers concluded that the Rhythm Method, although applicable for long periods of time by those women who had regular menstrual cycles, was bound eventually to fail, particularly during periods of stress or at the onset of irregularity before the menopause. The Temperature Method had the merit of identifying the time of ovulation in each cycle and was therefore independent of chance variations in cycle lengths. However, this information was supplied in retrospect so that only the late safe days of the luteal phase were identified and no information was provided on the many days of infertility which preceded ovulation. This deficiency was particularly serious in women with long irregular cycles, in lactating women and in women approaching the menopause. When I first met Dr. Billings and Father Catarinich in 1963 and saw their data, I was most impressed by its extent and the thoroughness with which it had been appraised. They had hundreds of temperature charts showing every type of normal and abnormal menstrual cycle which had only recently been documented by laborious hormone assays on a few women. They had records extending for years on individual women as they approached the menopause, in an attempt to identify subtle changes which might indicate recommencement of ovarian activity after months of amenorrhea. They had tested every possible method of defining the temperature shift and had tried every possible rule for determining when intercourse could be safely resumed in an effort to decrease the failure rates. By 1963 they had concluded that neither the Rhythm Method nor the Temperature Method, nor a combination of the two could provide an accepted degree of safety in return for the restrictions imposed. The methods were inelegant because they did not identify the majority of the days of infertility which the couple could be using for intercourse. Therefore, they began to investigate the possible use of cervical mucus as an indicator of the days of fertility and infertility. This symptom was already well recognized by gynecologists and endocrinologists, but the question was whether it could be identified with reliability by the women themselves. It was at this stage that Dr. Lyn Billings became an essential member of the team. She, together with her female colleagues, found that they could describe in minute detail the cyclical changes in mucus secretions and in the sensations they felt in the vaginal area, and showed that these changes were closely related to the underlying ovarian activity. From then on the Ovulation Method became exclusively a woman's preserve, and men were relegated to the position of observers, a very important and often resented change in roles compared with most other forms of contraception.

At first, the women correlated their mucous symptoms with their previous experience gained from the Rhythm calculations and the Temperature records. However, it was soon realized that the new method was probably considerably superior to the others and that more accurate markers were required for comparison. Therefore, Dr. Henry Burger and I were asked to test the accuracy of the mucous symptoms against the available hormone markers of ovulation, namely the midcycle peaks of serum and urinary LH, FSH and estrogen and the rise in progesterone production. These hormone markers were then correlated with the exact time of ovulation as determined by direct visualization of the ovaries at laparoscopy or laparotomy. With this secure basis, the women were then able to refine still further their descriptions of the mucous symptoms which were associated with the fertile and infertile phases of the cycle and with ovulation. These mucous symptoms were not identical for every woman and at first it was thought that only about 70 percent of women would be able to recognize them. However, with experience and the assurance provided by the hormone assays, it was shown that all fertile women have recognizable symptoms. A stated absence of symptoms is due either to inexperience of the observer or to a state of infertility. These studies produced an enormous amount of data on hormone values, mucous symptoms and temperature records under all possible conditions of normal and abnormal ovarian activity. This is by far the largest hormonal study of reproduction in the human female yet performed. The data have been so extensive that they have saturated the publication facilities of the two laboratories and consequently only a fraction has reached the scientific journals. Some is presented by Mercedes Wilson in this book.

The figures and statistics required by the scientific community seem irrelevant and unimportant. The following story illustrates the problem. In 1976, the analysis of the hormone values and mucous symptoms in 104 normal menstrual cycles had been completed and we were discussing progress over dinner. Drs. John and Lyn Billings, Father Catarinich, Dr. Pat Harrisson and I were present. Dr. Lyn Billings then introduced her latest concept concerning the basic infertile mucous pattern, which persists day after day and signifies continuing infertility. It was a brilliant concept because it changed the emphasis from the recognition of the fertile days to that of the much more numerous infertile days. Furthermore, once stated it was an obvious truth because fertility and ovulation depend on cyclical events and a steady state must necessarily be infertile. The concept required verification by hormone analyses. Thus it was agreed that 25 trained volunteers would contribute daily specimens for a complete cycle during which they recorded their mucous symptoms. The aim was to correlate the first change from the postmenstrual mucous pattern with the first rise in estrogen output. At the same time the study would provide the best possible figures relating the last day of fertile type mucus (Peak day) with the day of ovulation, using the latest refinements in the Ovulation Method. The women went to work with enthusiasm to recruit volunteers. No more than a week later, Dr. Meg Smith, who runs the laboratory, came into my office to check on details. Twenty-five women had been agreed upon, more than 30 were already collecting with more to come! Two weeks later she reported that two of the volunteers had just returned from Europe and were having the most complicated mucous patterns they had ever recorded, another had volunteered because of difficult mucous patterns and was having an anovulatory cycle, and at least five others had volunteered because they were having difficulty in becoming pregnant and were hoping that the hormone values would help them. So much for our plans for a perfect study!

During the early days of the Ovulation Method, the women were taught to use the mucous symptoms in conjunction with the temperature records and the rhythm calculations. The problem inevitably arose as to which to believe when discrepancies occurred between the different observations. Dr. Lyn Billings took the bold step of stating that the mucous symptoms were the most correct, and as the temperature record and calendar calculations were confusing the picture, they should be abandoned altogether except in special cases. Thus the Ovulation Method in its present form came into existence. The laboratory investigations had by then demonstrated that the Peak symptom (last day of fertile type mucus) was as accurate in dating ovulation as any of the hormone markers, and that the temperature shift was the least reliable of the indices used in this study. Furthermore, the hormone studies had confirmed that the fertile type mucus was caused by the high preovulatory estrogen values, and had also shown that the sudden change to infertile type mucus which followed the Peak day was caused by the rise in progesterone secretion at this time rather than by the fall in estrogen production. Thus the Peak day phenomenon was caused by the same rise in progesterone which caused the temperature shift and was a more sensitive indicator of this event. The decision to dispense with the thermometer and rhythm calculations caused a bitter division amongst natural family planners, so that today two main methods are employed, the Symptothermal Method and the Ovulation Method (Billings) which forms the subject of this book.

With a world-wide demand for improved natural methods of family planning, the Ovulation Method introduced in Australia in the 1950s, spread and was quickly accepted in other countries. It attracted some brilliant supporters, including Mercedes Wilson, who introduced the system of charts and stamps which have become almost the symbols of the Ovulation Method itself. Others in developing countries have introduced new teaching aids for nonliterate people. Nevertheless, attempts to improve the Method continue, and it is necessary that the process which led to the development of the Ovulation Method, namely the detailed appraisal of all unplanned pregnancies, must go on. This process of continual modification of the rules, both by the originators and by others throughout the world in an attempt to entirely eliminate unplanned pregnancies, has led to much confusion. Thus the continual updating of the *Atlas of the Ovulation Method* published from Melbourne has been necessary. The chief purpose of the present book is to present the Ovulation Method as the author sees it in the late seventies and in the eighties; and in this she provides a most valued service. The book is profusely illustrated and contains the most comprehensive collection of stamp charts compiled by women of many different countries illustrating the universal application of the Ovulation Method. Chapters are included on the underlying processes involved in reproduction and on the scientific findings which relate these processes to the mucous symptoms. An evaluation of the user-effectiveness of the Ovulation Method and of methods of family planning in general are also covered.

The world-wide dissemination of the Ovulation Method has raced ahead of the facilities for publishing the scientific basis of the Method. This has led to the criticism that the Method has been promoted more by religious zeal than by scientific merit. It is hoped that this criticism will be allayed when all the hormone studies are finally published in scientific journals. Nevertheless, reliable figures for the user-effectiveness of the Method as practised in 1978 have yet to be obtained. It is obvious that methods of natural family planning are, of all methods, most open to user failure because of the need for complete abstinence over the fertile period. This demands complete communication and cooperation between husband and wife. It is for this reason that the Natural Family Planning Associations are mainly religion-based and are very much involved in marriage guidance. It must be understood that the cooperation and understanding between partners which are essential for applying the natural methods are beneficial to the marriage as a whole. It should be emphasized that any attempt at sexual contact using withdrawal or mechanical contraception during the fertile phase distorts the mucous symptoms, causing errors in interpretation at this most crucial time. Furthermore, our hormone studies suggest that intercourse *during the fertile period* may advance ovulation and thus shorten the period of safety provided by the rules.

Accurate figures on the degree of method reliability if the rules are adhered to are of prime importance to the couple. Mercedes Wilson attempts to answer this, but agrees that more extensive studies are required. There is a tendency for witch hunts to be started by every unplanned pregnancy. Yet all methods of contraception have failure rates, and the real question is whether these are acceptable for the advantages gained. Mercedes Wilson in the chapter on user-effectiveness shows that, as for other methods of family planning, motivation of the couple is most important. The failure rate of the Ovulation Method is much higher for those who are spacing their families than for those whose families are completed. The WHO is conducting trials on the effectiveness of the Ovulation Method in several countries. The results are awaited with much interest. Preliminary results indicate that the majority of the failures have occurred during the first few months of the trials and that thereafter the performance of the Method is remarkably good with completely acceptable failure rates. Whether this trend is due to the early elimination of the most highly fertile couples or to increasing experience in the recognition of the mucous symptoms is not yet determined.

Our results are based on 70 complete cycles from 54 normally ovulating women studied daily with hormone assays (serum/urine LH, urine estrogen and urine pregnanediol), with mucous symptoms and temperature records. We have also studied 43 women post-partum and during breast feeding; these have been studied by urine assays on a weekly basis, together with mucous symptoms, for a total of 390 months (average of 9 months per subject). Eighty-three pre-menopausal women have been studied daily or weekly with mucous symptoms for 1 month. Two pre-menopausal women have been studied weekly at intervals for 5–7 years; a total of 63 months have been studied in these two patients. Two girls have been studied as they passed through menarche and first ovulation from the ages of 11–16 years—these were mainly weekly assays, giving a total of 60 months studied.

In the normally ovulating women full data were available in 66 cycles, in which the last day of fertile mucus was able to be correlated with the LH peak, which is considered to occur approximately 17 hours before ovulation. In 56 cycles (85%) the last day of fertile mucus (Peak symptom) occurred within ± 1 day of the LH peak; however, when considering our assessment of the time of ovulation by the LH peak it should be remembered that this can be in error by 1 day in approximately 20% of cycles.

This book by Mercedes Wilson is a most valuable addition to the literature on the Ovulation Method. It will do much to educate potential users in the current application of the Method and will give them the necessary confidence in applying it. She is to be congratulated for a fine effort.

JAMES B. BROWN, D.Sc., Ph.D.,
Professor, Department of Obstetrics & Gynaecology,
University of Melbourne, Australia;
Professor, Department of OB-GYN,
Royal Women's Hospital, Melbourne, Australia.

Acknowledgments

I would like to express my appreciation to the many people who helped me to write this book:

- To Dr. John Billings and Dr. Evelyn Billings, of Melbourne, Australia, who originated the Ovulation Method and helped spread it throughout the world;
- To Dr. James Brown, professor, Department of Obstetrics and Gynaecology at Melbourne University, who worked over 5,000 hormonal correlations that scientifically support the Ovulation Method and who provided much of the scientific information for Chapter 2;
- To Dr. John Casey, of Sydney, Australia, who provided the results of his study, "Correlation of Mid-cycle Mucus and Ovulation", for Chapter 2;
- To Dr. Thomas Hilgers, of Omaha, Nebraska, who contributed data of his latest research for Chapter 2;
- To Dr. Kevin Hume, who contributed much information to Chapter 8 and advised me while I wrote the rest of the book;
- To Dr. John J. Brennan, who continues to give generously of his time and efforts to spread the knowledge of the Ovulation Method not only in the United States, but also to Latin America;
- To Dr. Herb Ratner, who contributed valuable information to Chapter 8;
- To Dr. Janis Dunlap, of Tulane University, who contributed Chapter 2;
- To Dr. Joan King, who helped me through various chapters of the book and whose advice I greatly value;
- To Dr. Mark Ordy, of Tulane University's Delta Primate Center, who helped revise the manuscript, and to his assistants, Pamela Medart and Robbie Sharp;
- To Dr. Jay Hansche, who contributed Chapter 11 on the statistical Evaluation of Contraceptive techniques.
- To Mr. Angus Brown, of Wharton, Texas, whose editing and advice guided me through every chapter;
- To Dr. Walker Percy, whose editing and encouragement guided me through to the end of the book;
- To Mrs. Jane Mueller, my medical editor, whose advice and editing work enhanced the clarity of this book;
- To Dr. Leo O'Gorman, whose advice I greatly appreciate;
- To Mr. Ringold Olivier, who spent hundreds of hours working on the charts and

other parts of the manuscript, and provided continuous support throughout the writing of this book;

• To the missionaries and to the women everywhere who sent information that was analyzed and incorporated into this book;

• To Father William Gibbons, M.D. of El Salvador, to Sister Francisca Kearns, and to Father Denis St. Marie of Guatemala, whose unceasing work on the Ovulation Method in Latin America has set a fine example of future missionaries engaged in pastoral work;

• To Father Manuel Rodriguez and to Bishop Miguel Rodriguez, and to Mrs. Ana Oriol de Ruiz and Mrs. Alva Nazario de Fantauzzi, who have helped the Ovulation Method succeed in Puerto Rico;

• To Father Rached, of the Dominican Republic, to Sister Byrne and Sister McEwen, of Korea, to Sister Lucille Levasseur, of Fiji, and Sister Mary Pittman and Sister Adriane, of New Guinea. Their work inspired me to write Chapter 10;

• To Mrs. Sylvia de Jaramillo, of Mexico, and to Miss Sheila McShane, of Guatemala;

• To Sister Catherine Bernard, M.D., of India, who supplied charts and other information, and to Sister Leoni McSweeney, M.D. of Nigeria;

• To all the teachers in the United States who give their time to help families learn the Ovulation Method;

• To the regional coordinators: Mrs. Rita Ayd of Maryland, Sister Anne Boessen of Illinois, Dr. John Brennan of Wisconsin, Mrs. Kathryn Claiborne of North Carolina, Mrs. Lou Paula Egenolf of Texas, Mrs. Kay Ek of Minnesota, Mrs. Mary Lee Fiegel and Mr. and Mrs. Tom Ford of Wisconsin, Mrs. Marilyn Grover of Oregon, Mrs. Marge Harrigan and Mr. John Foley of Texas, Dr. Howard Herning of California, Mrs. Nancy Fisher, RN of Florida, Mrs. Leah Jackson of Massachusetts, Mr. and Mrs. Don Kramer of Minnesota, Mrs. Maureen Liberto of Mississippi, Mr. and Mrs. Jose Maes of California, Mrs. Margaret McGauley of Missouri, Mrs. Marian Ruth of Michigan, Mrs. Alida Smith of Georgia, Mr. and Mrs. Dennis Doherty of Wyoming, and Mrs. Ann Walsh of California.

• To Mrs. Judy Ford, of Covington, who helped develop the teaching charts, and to Mrs. Margot Koch and Mrs. Gerry Mellerine, who became substitute teachers to give me time to write the book; and to Mrs. Rosi Young.

• To my former secretary, Mrs. Peggy Thompson, and to Mrs. Delaine Yates, who devoted themselves to the book, and to Miss Betsy Law, who typed the final draft of the manuscript;

• To the officials of the De Rance Foundation of Milwaukee, Wis., which paid all of my office expenses while I wrote the book.

• Findings cited in the text and/or in the appendices are being published with the permission of the authors and publishers.

Contents

Appendices

1

An Overview

The purpose of this book is to make women more aware of their own fertility by learning to recognize and use to their advantage signs of fertile and infertile phases of their menstrual cycles. This knowledge will empower them to control their fertility, to conceive or to avoid conception. The ongoing knowledge resulting from widespread use of the natural method of birth control has made it possible to offer an alternative to the use of artificial methods.

Results of studies about the reliability of this natural method together with its unlimited availability suggest an effective, unique way for women of all persuasions to control fertility without health risks, ranging from those who prefer nature's way to those who are guided by religious principles. Setting aside the concern about side effects and unknown future consequences, the greatest harm resulting from the expedient use of contraceptives and intrauterine devices may be that they hinder exploration of safer alternative methods based on increasing scientific knowledge about human reproduction.

The Ovulation Method of Natural Family Planning was developed by Dr. John Billings of Melbourne, Australia. His research on natural family planning started 25 years ago, and in the course of the years developed the Ovulation Method which is the most promising natural method available in the world today. It must not be confused with the Rhythm Method nor with the Temperature Method. It is simply based on a woman's recognition of the changes in her own cervical mucus secreted a few days before, and during the time of ovulation. This ability to determine the period of fertility gives the couple the freedom to achieve or postpone pregnancy without intrusion of drugs or mechanical devices of any kind.

The Ovulation Method approach has great potential since a woman can use it diligently with the assurance that "she is working with nature," rather than using drugs or other devices to interfere with an exceedingly complex and delicate biological clock.

Men and women should not be put off by the challenge of controlling their natural fertility by natural methods. (The ability to reproduce, a wondrous capability to be treasured, must also be directed and regulated.) We should accept the responsibilities that come with our freedom of choice to select the most effective and least harmful methods of regulating births.

By 1945, there was an increasing awareness of, and great publicity concerning, the population explosion, particularly in developing countries. In the United States and other technologically advanced countries, there was the "baby boom" after World War II. Due in part to the alarming increase in world population, there was increasing political, cultural, and economic urgency to develop a simple, safe and economic contraceptive method to be used in both technologically advanced and developing countries. By 1950 scientists had established that hormones could prevent ovulation in animals. From 1950 to 1960, much research was done into the biochemistry of steroid hormones, particularly the sex hormones. By 1960, a compound consisting of a combination of synthetic progesterone and estrogen was approved as an oral contraceptive in the United States. It soon became known throughout the world as the Pill. Since 1960, proponents of the Pill have made it attractive to women by proposing that it is the most effective, convenient and reversible contraceptive that has ever been devised. The Pill has been given credit for declining birth rates, and a wide range of social changes and improvements, particularly in the status of women.

Although the Pill still is one of the most popular contraceptives, an increasing number of clinical studies have reported various adverse side effects, and contraindications. Scientists have established that hormones are some of the most potent modifiers of the biochemistry and physiology of the body. As a result, considerable skepticism has arisen concerning the wisdom of administering the potent hormone compounds that the Pill contains, to healthy women for long periods of time, when the ultimate effects of the health of the women are unknown. Hormones affect the metabolism of virtually every cell in the body. There is considerable evidence that the Pill abolishes not only the normal fertility cycle in women but that it alters normal metabolism, and may have various side effects as well as cause some serious disorders, particularly when administered for extended periods of time. In view of the undetermined effects of gonadal hormones and contraceptive steroids on metabolism, it is becoming apparent that none of the currently available oral contraceptives are as safe and effective as it had originally been hoped (Seaman and Seaman 1977).

The spectacular advances in science have invited reliance on the use of an increasing number of drugs, including those used for birth control. The U.S. Government spends $366 million each year for all forms of contraception throughout the world, but less than $1 million on natural methods of family planning (Kane 1977). People have resorted first to what has been readily available and heavily promoted by government and industry—artificial contraceptives. With the increasing number of adverse reports concerning side effects and unknown risks involved in the prolonged use of the Pill, many women are taking greater responsibility for their own health.

Despite the absence of government funding, the Ovulation Method has spread to more than 80 countries in less than a decade. The teaching has been done by volunteers and it has been supported by donations from private persons.

2

The Female Reproductive System, Ovulation, Cervical Mucous Secretion

Since the Ovulation Method requires a woman to learn to recognize the internal changes in her body related to her procreative potential, the practitioner of this method usually has more than a casual interest in what these internal changes represent, and how they take place. Sexual reproduction, the union of sperm from the male with the ovum from the female, ensures the biological survival of man as a species. Yet this union of ovum and sperm can only occur during a few crucial days of the normal ovulation cycle. The average length of the healthy female's ovulatory cycle is approximately 28 days. However, cycle length may vary considerably from woman to woman, and in an individual woman the cycle length may vary widely. Further, after the onset of menstruation (menarche), and also when a woman is nearing the menopause, cycles are often irregular and anovulatory. The existence of a cycle, however, is a necessary prerequisite to a functioning reproductive system and to fertility. The topic of this chapter is the complex interplay of internal secretions within a female that determine the ovulatory cycle. The most important organs of secretion are: (1) the brain, which is connected by nerves and by vascular channels to a gland; (2) the pituitary gland, which controls the sexual organs; (3) the ovaries. The anatomical relationship of these organs is illustrated in Figure 2–1.

As shown in Figure 2–1, the brain interacts with the pituitary gland through the hypothalamus. Although crucial in the control of such essential bodily functions as eating, drinking and sleeping, this small area at the ventral surface of the brain is particularly important in the control of the female's sexual cycle. In women, the hypothalamus senses the current state of the cycle mainly through the circulating levels of the two ovarian hormones estradiol and progesterone, and controls the pituitary gland by a hormone, gonadotropin releasing hormone (Gn-RH), which is frequently called luteinizing hormone releasing hormone (LH-RH). This hypothalamic releasing hormone is synthesized within the neurons and transfers information within the nervous system to the reproductive system. At the junction of brain and pituitary, impulses of the brain are translated into signals turning the reproductive organs on or

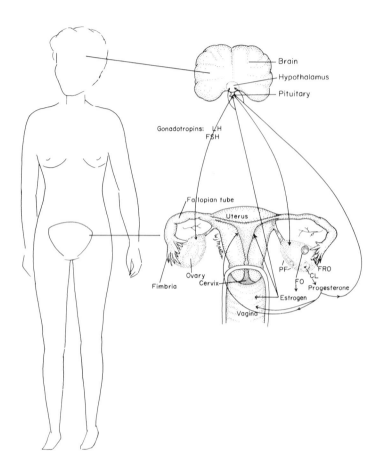

Figure 2–1. Anatomy and physiology of the adult female reproductive system.

off. Although there are no nerve connections between the hypothalamus and the anterior pituitary, there are numerous vascular bridges. At the base of the brain these specialized blood vessels are in close contact with nerve cells and the hypothalamic hormone is released from the nerve cells into the blood. The vessels aggregate and drain into the anterior or front portion of the pituitary where the hypothalamic hormone now comes in contact with gonadotropin-producing cells in the pituitary. In this manner the brain modifies the activity of the anterior pituitary gland.

In response to hormonal signals from the hypothalamus the anterior pituitary releases various amounts of two hormones—gonadotropins—that control the female cycle. The first of these gonadotropins, follicle stimulating hormone, (FSH), causes structures in the ovary to grow into ovum-containing organs called follicles. While under the influence of FSH and while growing rapidly, the follicle releases a hormone called estrogen, which causes many of the changes in the accessory organs of reproduction, e.g. cervical mucus, of which much more will be said later. The second pituitary hormone, luteinizing hormone (LH), plays its most important role after the follicle in the ovary has matured its ovum. The process of folliculogenesis requires a period of raised FSH secretion by the pituitary which causes the ovarian follicle to grow and mature, migrate to the surface of the ovary, and finally, under the influence of LH, burst, (ovulation), releasing the ovum into a funnel-like opening at the end of the fallopian tubes, called the fimbria (see Figure 2–1). The ovum is swept into the fallopian tubes by tiny hairlike projections from the inside of the fimbria and is propelled down the fallopian tubes until it reaches the uterus. Meanwhile the second pituitary hormone, LH, which peaks at the time of ovulation and causes the release of the ovum, produces a transmutation of the empty follicle which develops into the corpus luteum, or "yellow body," that secretes, in addition to estradiol, another hormone, progesterone. Progesterone is necessary for the survival of the embryo in the uterus if the ovum is fertilized by a male sperm. Progesterone also causes the abrupt change from fertile to infertile type mucus, seen immediately after ovulation. The combination of high levels of progesterone and estrogen suppresses the secretion of FSH and prevents the further development of new follicles and thus prevents the next ovum from being matured. Typically, only one follicle, the dominant one, will ovulate during one cycle. Other follicles approaching maturity during a particular cycle assist by secreting small amounts of estrogen, but when ovulation of the dominant follicle occurs, these lesser follicles become atretic and regress.

In discussing cyclical changes it is customary to date events from the first day bleeding occurs. The first half of a menstrual cycle is called the follicular or proliferative stage, since it involves developing the primitive follicle in response to the secretion of the pituitary gonadotropin, FSH; and as the follicle grows, it secretes estrogen which causes proliferative changes in the uterus and vagina. After the estrogen peak and LH surge produce ovulation, the second half of the cycle is referred to as the luteal or secretory phase since the corpus luteum secretes progesterone which causes the endometrial lining of the uterus to develop many sawtooth-shaped secreting glands. If fertilization and implantation of the ovum do not occur, the corpus luteum degenerates by day 26 in a cycle of 28 days and progesterone secretion ceases. With the withdrawal of both estrogen and progesterone, the endometrial lining of the uterus and thickened vaginal lining diminish in size, blood vessels become blocked, and tissues deprived of oxygen decay and fall away in menstruation. The bleeding surface is repaired as estrogen from new follicles begins to be secreted by the ovary due to FSH release from the pituitary in response to the signal from the hypothalamus. Thus, another ovulation cycle begins. If the ovulated ovum is fertilized, the developing embryo secretes a new hormone, human chorionic gonadotropin (HCG), which has many of the properties of pituitary LH. This causes the corpus luteum to grow for several months and secrete the progesterone necessary for maintaining the pregnancy. Therefore the uterine lining is not sloughed away, and a new ovulation cycle does not commence. These sequences of uterine, ovarian, and pituitary events during a normal cycle are shown in Figure 2–2.

The above description presents the main components of the cyclical control of ovulation, fertility and menstruation. But the complex hormonal interrelations, feedback systems, and neural control of this intricate process are still incompletely understood and are the subject of much research today.

A discussion of one of the more obvious aspects of hormonal control of the woman's reproductive system, the Pill, is covered in Chapter 8. In the present context, it is necessary to mention only that in general, oral contraceptives act by inhib-

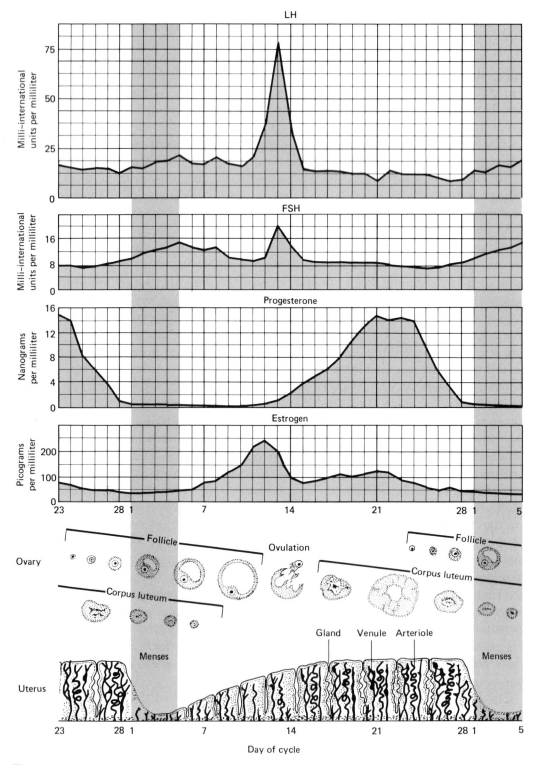

Figure 2–2. Scheme of the endometrial and ovarian events in a normal menstrual cycle. (Permission of Scientific American)

iting ovulation. This is achieved by simulating the high estrogen and progesterone levels during the luteal phase of the menstrual cycle just described. As will be shown later, progesterone has a powerful inhibitory effect on the production of fertile type cervical mucus. This fertile type mucus is necessary for the sperm deposited in the vagina at intercourse to migrate through the cervix to reach the egg. Normally progesterone production is very low in the preovulatory period. However, progestogen provided by oral contraceptives given early in the cycle produces an abnormal state in which fertile type mucus is prevented from being formed. This is a potent contraceptive action.

Approximately 500,000 potential follicles are present in a female's ovary at birth. Of these potential follicles, only 300 to 400 will ovulate during the woman's reproductively fertile life. The human female in our society usually becomes sexually mature and capable of bearing children at about 14 years of age, although sexual maturity may occur earlier. Ova are released periodically for years until cycling finally ceases at menopause. The age span during which a woman may conceive ranges from approximately 14 to 50 years in the United States. Throughout the span of life, the rhythmic cycles of internal change within the ovaries are accompanied by external changes that can be sensed by the woman taught to recognize them. The external symptoms of ovarian activity which a woman can recognize during a 28-day normal cycle not terminating in pregnancy are 3 to 7 days of bleeding or menstruation during days 1 to 7, fertile type cervical mucous discharges from days 10 to 15, followed by a sudden change to infertile type mucus which persists from days 16 to 25, and then some symptoms of premenstrual bloating, tension or breast tenderness. In the first 2 to 3 days of menstruation the upper two-thirds of the endometrium are sloughed away. In the next 2 to 3 days of menstruation, the bleeding surface is repaired. By day 12, the follicle is approaching maturity and the ovum is released on day 14 in response to pituitary stimulation. If the ovum is not fertilized during days 13, 14, or 15, the corpus luteum degenerates by day 26.

The most obvious external sign of ovarian activity is, of course, menstruation. However, ovulation is the most important event in the reproductive cycle and as shown in the above sequence occurs approximately 10 to 14 days prior to menstrual bleeding. It is necessary, therefore, to recognize the signs and symptoms of ovulation if control is to be achieved over the reproductive process. The most important of these signs is the change in the consistency of cervical mucus produced by the peak in estrogen, released by the follicle during its rapid stage of growth prior to ovulation, followed by the rise in progesterone which occurs immediately after ovulation.

The cervix measures approximately 2 to 4 cm in length and is a continuation of the lower portion of the uterus. The epithelium of the endocervical canal is characterized by tall, columnar secretory cells. Cell size and the amount of secretions of the endocervical cells are cyclical. They vary according to stimulation by ovarian estrogen. The size of the cells is greatest at the time of ovulation when the concentration of circulating estrogen is highest. The cervical mucus is most copious and the viscosity is markedly decreased during the 1 to 2 days immediately preceding ovulation. In noticeable contrast, during the intermediate postmenstrual phase and during the luteal phase, the amount of mucus is less and is of different viscosity. The changing characteristics of cervical mucus secretions from preovulatory day 10 through ovulation on day 14 and the postovulatory days 15 through 28 will be described and illustrated in photographs in Chapter 3.

The glycoprotein filaments in the cervical mucous secretions are arranged so that the spaces between the meshwork of filaments measure approximately 2 to 5 microns while under the influence of estrogen. During the luteal phase, under the influence of progesterone, the spaces in the meshwork are reduced from approximately 2 microns to 0.5 microns. Since the size of the filament meshes is greatest around the time of ovulation, sperm can pass freely through the meshwork of the filaments and through the endocervical canal to reach the ovum. Scientists have correlated the sperm penetration of filaments with the amount, dry content and other characteristics of the mucous secretions. These relationships together with the changes in basal body temperature which occur during a typical 28-day cycle are shown in Figure 2–3.

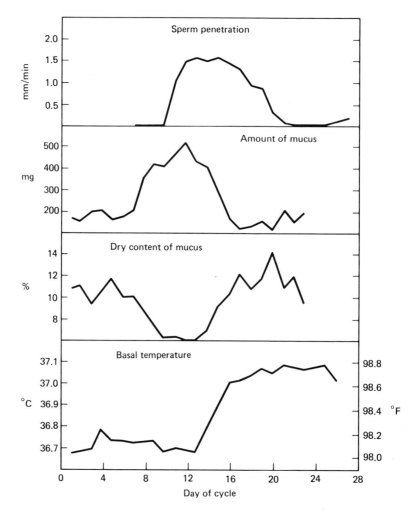

Figure 2–3. Correlation of sperm penetration, amount and dry content of mucous secretion and basal body temperature in relation to the average 28-day reproductive cycle. (Permission from Bishop, D.N.: In Young, N.C., editor: Sex and Internal Secretions, vol. 2, ed. 3, Baltimore, 1961, the Williams & Wilkins Co.)

P.H.

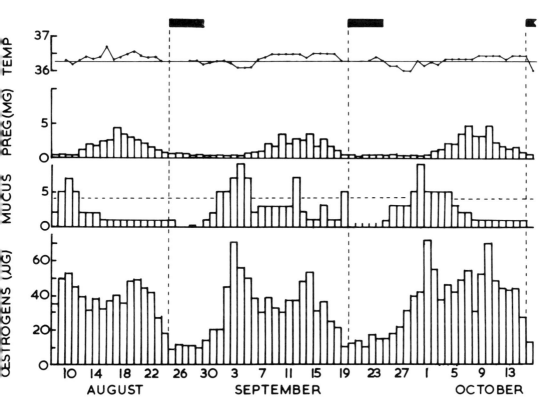

Figure 2–4. Urinary estrogen and pregnanediol values, mucous symptoms and basal temperature during three cycles in a normal subject. (Brown, J.B., 1978)

It is not unusual for the "average" cycle described above to become disrupted by environmental or psychological events. Stimuli arising from external events are sensed by the brain and may influence sexual cyclicity via the hypothalamus. It is through this mechanism that times of severe physical or emotional stress, or disease can influence a woman's periodicity. These occurrences will be described in detail in Chapter 7. Relative to the current chapter, however, one should consider what happens, for example, if the pattern of FSH-Estrogen-LH feedback sequence is not "normal". The major variability in a woman's cycle occurs in the preovulatory stage of the cycle. If FSH secretion, for whatever reason, does not rise rapidly to high enough levels to cause full follicular growth, ovulation will be delayed. A woman's mucous symptoms will alert her to this arrested cycle. Once ovulation occurs, the remainder of the cycle proceeds with little variability between cycles and between women, in that bleeding occurs 10 to 14 days later.

The relationship between the patterns of cervical mucous secretion and the amounts of estrogen and progesterone secreted by the ovaries as measured by the excretion of estrogens and pregnanediol in urine, has been studied extensively (Brown, 1978). His conclusions are based on over 700 cycles from more than 50 different women with regular menstrual cycles and of proven fertility, in more than 40 lactating women, and in more than 80 premenopausal women. Representative examples of the cyclic variation in estrogen and progesterone in a variety of different menstrual cycles are presented in Figures 2–4 to 2–13. A close correlation was demonstrated under all conditions between the hormone values and the mucous symptoms. The start of the period of possible fertility was identified by the first appearance of mucus, and this was closely correlated with the first rise in urinary estrogens. Figure 2–4 shows daily urinary estrogen and pregnanediol values during 3 consecutive normal ovulatory cycles from one individual. The mucus was rated on a scale of –1 (dry) to +9 (maximally fertile). Any value of 5 and above corresponded to the category of fertile type mucus. The estrogen values rose steadily prior to ovulation as the follicle matured under the influence of FSH secretion. The maximum mucous symptoms and highest estrogen values practically coincided during each of the 3 cycles. Peak day of mucous secretion is defined as the last day of fertile type mucus. Notice that the decline in estrogen values after the peak was relatively rapid; however, the rapid change in the mucous symptom at this time was more the result of the rising progesterone production which overrides the estrogen effect. After the peak in estrogen values and mucous symptoms, the progesterone levels as indicated by the urinary pregnanediol values rose due to the secretory activity of the corpus luteum.

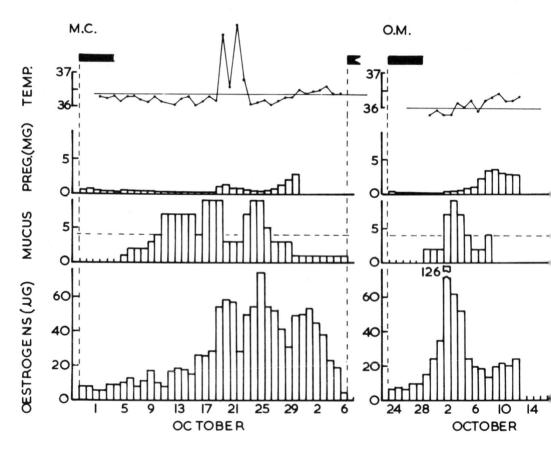

Figure 2–5. Urinary estrogen and pregnanediol values, mucous symptoms and basal temperature in a cycle with a double mid-cycle estrogen peak. (Brown, J.B., 1978)

The pregnanediol levels remained high until several days before onset of bleeding. When progesterone secretion is elevated, the mucus is typically of the nonfertile type. The basal body temperature provides another index of ovulation and subsequent progesterone secretion, and is shown at the top of Figure 2-4. Progesterone is thermogenic and the body temperature rises as the pregnanediol values increase, and provides an independent marker that ovulation has occurred. However, in all these studies it was apparent that there was less consistency in the relation between the rise in temperature and the rise in progesterone than was observed between the mucous symptoms, the estrogen peak and the subsequent rise in pregnanediol values. As shown in Figure 2-4, the estrogen values fall after the preovulatory peak and then rise again to a second maximum which occurs about the time of the maximum pregnanediol values. Thereafter, both estrogen and pregnanediol values fall and menstruation ensues. During the second estrogen maximum, the mucous symptoms are suppressed by the raised progesterone values at this time. A deviation from this pattern is shown in Figure 2-5. Notice that in this cycle the first estrogen peak was followed by only a small rise in pregnanediol excretion, thus showing that ovulation did not occur at this time. A second estrogen peak occurred 5 days later and was followed by a postovulatory rise in pregnanediol excretion and basal temperature. Mucous peaks coincided with both estrogen peaks in this case, and ovulation followed the second peak in estrogen excretion. In this particular case, a severe infection was experienced (note the high temperature at the time of the first estrogen peak, when ovulation should have occurred) about the time of expected ovulation. Ovulation was delayed and mucus regressed. The second peak in estrogen and mucus occurred 4 to 5 days later, followed by ovulation and a subsequent pregnanediol rise. This example is illustrative of the accuracy in charting mucous symptoms to determine fertility. Especially when infection or disease is apparent, ovulation may be delayed. Mucus alerts the woman to this fact.

Figure 2-6 illustrates one type of anovulatory cycle in which there is an estrogen peak but no subsequent rise in pregnanediol and estrogen excretion showing that ovulation did not occur. The estrogen values have been separated into three estrogens; estriol, estrone, and estradiol. During such cycles, patches of fertile type mucus are observed corresponding to the raised estrogen values, but there is no sharp cut-off because there is no rise in progesterone production and fertile type mucus is observed almost up to the time of menstrual bleeding. The lack of a definite Peak day symptom indicates lack of ovulation just as absence of progesterone reflects lack of ovulation.

A second type of anovulatory cycle is presented in Figure 2-7. Here the estrogen levels remained elevated and relatively constant between the first two episodes of bleeding. The second bleed occurred as a breakthrough phenomenon. This situation is produced when the FSH levels are not quite high enough to boost a follicle into an ovulatory response. When the estrogen has acted long enough to cause sufficient endometrial growth in the uterus, breakthrough bleeding or spotting occurs. The second episode of bleeding shown was followed by a peak in estrogen excretion which was followed by ovulation. This is a common cause of midcycle bleeding. Figure 2-8 illustrates another ovulatory cycle which ended in breakthrough bleeding. Fertile type mucus was not recorded until the estrogen values exceeded 10 ug/24 hrs, the

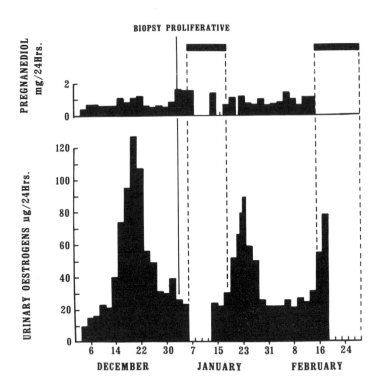

Figure 2–6. Urinary estrogens and pregnanediol values in anovulatory cycles with fluctuating estrogen output. (Brown, J.B. and Matthew, 1962)

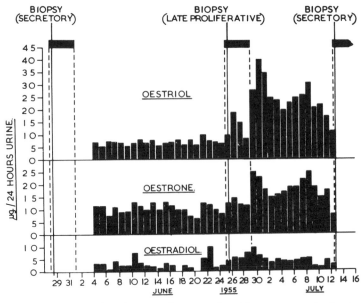

Figure 2–7. Urinary estrogen values in anovulatory cycle with constant raised estrogen excretion followed by ovulation and a normal luteal phase. (Brown and Matthew, 1962)

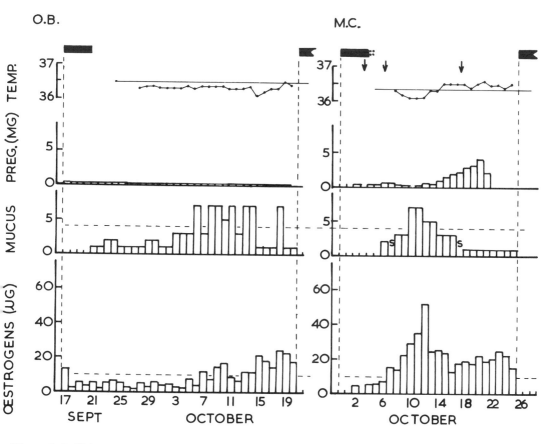

Figure 2-8. Urinary estrogen and pregnanediol values, mucous symptoms and basal temperature in an anovulatory cycle which ended in breakthrough bleeding. (Brown, 1978)

upper limit of estrogens derived from the adrenal glands, which is not sufficient to stimulate mucus production. In this type of anovulatory cycle, patches of fertile type cervical mucus occur at irregular and unpredictable intervals. It is of interest that a continuous mucous secretion is seldom seen as might be expected from the continuously elevated estrogen values in the presence of low pregnanediol values. It would appear that cervical production of mucus occurs in episodic bursts and thus resembles functionally many other endocrine organs.

Figure 2-9 shows a cycle with a prolonged follicular phase, lasting 28 days. Again fertile type mucus was not observed until the estrogen levels exceeded 10 ug/24 hrs and the event of ovulation on the 21st of October was verified by the subsequent rise in pregnanediol excretion. Brown suggests that such prolonged follicular phases are due to a delay in the rise of FSH. He maintains that in a normal cycle the pituitary secretion of FSH "hunts" upward seeking the threshold value required to evoke follicle growth. When the FSH values exceed this threshold, follicles begin to grow, but it takes several days before they are secreting the estrogen in sufficient concentrations to feed back to the hypothalamus to inhibit further FSH secretion from the pituitary. The FSH values rise still further to exceed an intermediate value before boosting the dominant follicle into an ovulatory response. Failure to exceed the threshold

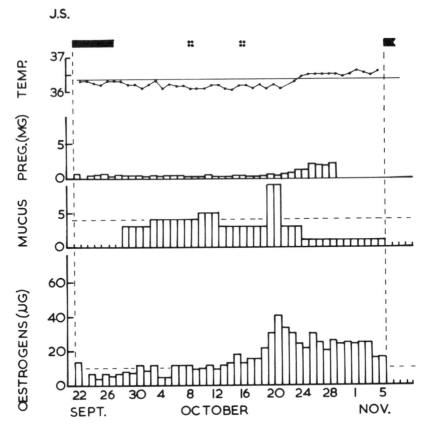

Figure 2-9. Urinary estrogen and pregnanediol values, mucous symptoms and basal temperature in a cycle with a prolonged follicular phase. (Brown, 1978)

leads to continued ovarian inactivity, and failure to exceed the intermediate level leads to the development of a group of follicles which secrete estrogen in constant amounts as occurs in the constant estrogen type of anovulatory cycle. Delay in the rise of FSH can cause one or both of these phenomena and thus lead to prolonged follicular phases as shown in Figures 2–7 and 2–8, and irregular appearances of fertile type mucus. In Figure 2–7, the FSH values finally exceeded the intermediate level and ovulation followed.

Figure 2–10 shows the estrogen and pregnanediol values in a woman immediately following childbirth and during lactation. Once again, the estrogen values are separated into three estrogens; estriol, estrone and estradiol. The low estrogen levels during lactation reflect a quiescent ovary and the absence of ovulation. About one month after lactation ceased, the estrogen levels began to rise in a cyclical manner and eventually reached a preovulatory peak 102 days after delivery. The cycle leading to the first bleed was ovulatory as judged by the pregnanediol values, but the luteal phase was abnormally short (7 days). The second cycle was ovulatory with a short luteal phase of 9 days duration, and the third cycle was the first in which the luteal phase was of normal duration and was thus potentially fertile. Short luteal phases are a common finding in ovulatory cycles which occur during lactation within 6 to 9 months of delivery.

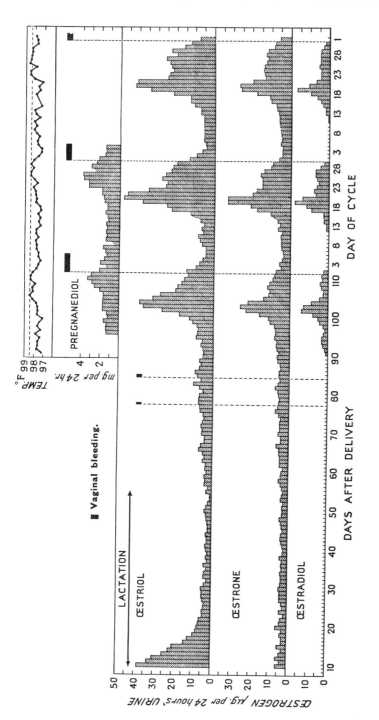

Figure 2–10. Urinary estrogen and pregnanediol values after delivery, during lactation, amenorrhea and the recommencement of normal ovarian activity. (Brown, 1956)

U.O. Breast feeding 18 months

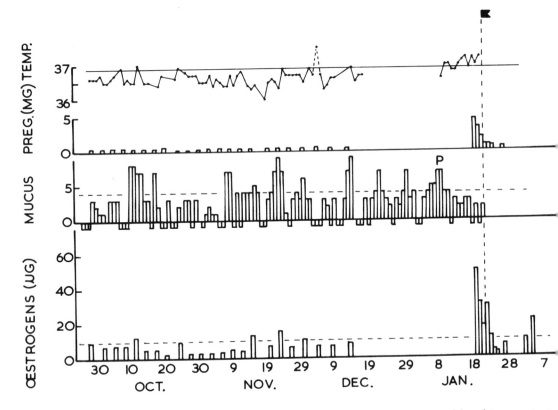

Figure 2–11. Urinary estrogen and pregnanediol values, mucous symptoms and basal temperature during lactation and the recommencement of normal ovarian activity. (Brown, 1978)

Figure 2–11 shows the results of a study commenced 18 months postpartum while the subject was still breast-feeding. Sporadic ovarian activity was evident at this time as judged by the sporadic increases in estrogen excretion above the level of 10 ug/24 hrs, the days of elevated estrogen corresponding closely with the appearances of fertile type mucus. The pregnanediol values remained uniformly low showing that ovulation was not occurring. During January, the subject observed ovulatory type mucus which was unmistakably like that seen before pregnancy, and therefore recommenced urine collections and basal temperature recording; her first bleed after pregnancy occurred 12 days later. An ovulatory cycle with completely normal characteristics was demonstrated by the estrogen and pregnanediol values, by the mucous symptoms and by the basal temperature record.

Figure 2–12 demonstrates the estrogen and pregnanediol values observed in a premenopausal woman over a period of 13 months. Hormone assays were performed weekly and mucous symptoms were recorded daily. Cycles were highly irregular with ovulatory cycles interspersed with anovulatory cycles. The study commenced during a period of 3 months amenorrhea; this ended in ovulation as shown by the rise in estrogen and pregnanediol values. The next two cycles were ovulatory. The cycle in February was anovulatory, of the fluctuating estrogen type. The next was an ovulatory cycle with a prolonged follicular phase. Ovulation also occurred during the May to June cycle. The next cycle was anovulatory of the fluctuating estrogen type, the July cycle was anovulatory of the constant estrogen type. The next cycle was prolonged and ended in ovulation, but a preovulatory breakthrough bleed occurred on 22nd September. The next two cycles were ovulatory. The subject recorded fertile type mucus with peak symptoms at the time of ovulation in all the ovulatory cycles except the last, and thus was able to recognize the times of possible fertility. A surprising feature was that during the anovulatory cycles, the mucous symptoms did not reflect some of the extremely high estrogen values seen, as might have been expected in the presence of the associated low pregnanediol values. The absence of fertile type mucus in the last ovulatory cycle recorded in December is explained by the elevated pregnanediol values which were seen during the preovulatory phase of this cycle. Such elevated preovulatory pregnanediol values are seen in some patients with infertility and it is unlikely that conception could have occurred during this cycle even though intercourse took place at time of ovulation. Thus despite her extreme irregularity, this subject was able to identify with considerable accuracy her times of possible fertility from her mucous symptoms. Practically all types of normal and abnormal ovarian activity were documented during the 13-month period.

The peak in urinary estrogen during a cycle, as the examples above illustrate, corresponds quite closely with the Peak day of mucous secretion. This estrogen peak occurs within 24 hours before the LH surge, and in most women ovulation occurs within 24 to 48 hours after the LH surge. It has been reported by Billings et al., (1972) that the average time between the Peak day of mucus and ovulation is 0.9 days. Thus, the determination of ovulation is accomplished retrospectively by an examination of the change in the mucus. After ovulation the mucus will abruptly change in consistency and color. This change in the mucus is due to the increase in ovarian progesterone as a consequence of corpus luteum activity. Figure 2–13 presents the relationship between LH surge, FSH peak, estrogen peak and pregnanediol (progesterone excretion) levels as detected by urinalysis and blood assays. Notice that FSH, LH, and estrogen peak around the time ovulation is assumed to occur. Progesterone, excreted as pregnanediol in the urine, remains at low levels preceding ovulation, but rises dramatically after ovulation.

Several laboratories, e.g. Flynn and Lynch (1976), Casey, (1977), Hilgers, Abraham and Cavanaugh (1978) using blood plasma analysis of steroids and gonadotropins have verified the close correlation between mucous symptoms and the hormonal accompaniments of ovulation during a normal fertile cycle. Figures 2–14 and 2–15 (from Casey, 1977) present serum levels of estradiol, progesterone and gonadotropins with corresponding mucus records superimposed. Blood was taken at 12-hour intervals and the time of ovulation was deduced from the hormonal changes. The follicular or preovulatory phase was considered to conclude with the day during which LH reached its peak, and the luteal or postovulatory phase was considered to commence on the day progesterone level exceeded 10 μmol/1. A remarkably close pattern of correspondence between these hormonal markers and mucus record is evident. Estradiol, FSH, and LH increase steadily and peak around the time of ovulation. Figure 2–14 is an example in which ovulation occurred 1 day following the day of peak mucus. This was the case in 7 out of 10 women studied. Fig-

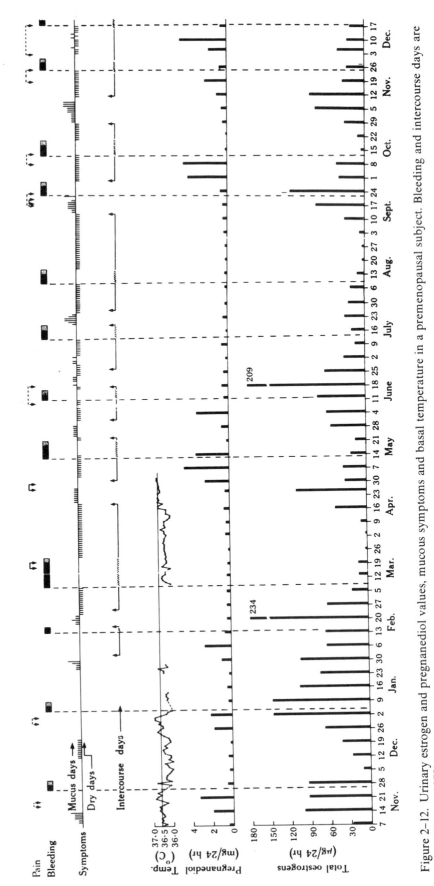

Figure 2–12. Urinary estrogen and pregnanediol values, mucous symptoms and basal temperature in a premenopausal subject. Bleeding and intercourse days are noted. (Brown, 1978)

ure 2–15 illustrates a case where the day of ovulation and the peak mucous symptom coincided. This occurred in 3 out of 10 women. These data are significant in showing the close relationship between ovulation and day of peak mucus. Since the human ovum remains viable for approximately 12 hours, the time of potential fertility is very transient, yet it would seem to be recognized with ease and accuracy using mucous symptoms.

In Figure 2–16 (from Hilgers, et al., 1978), which shows mean serum progesterone, LH, estradiol, basal body temperature and day of Peak symptom, the mean estimated time of ovulation in 65 normal ovulatory cycles occurred on average 0.31 days before the peak symptom. In this study, the time of ovulation was deduced from the level of progesterone. In 95.4 percent of the cycles, ovulation was estimated to occur from 2 days before, to 2 days after the peak symptom and the beginning of the mucous symptom preceded the estimated time of ovulation by an average of 5.9 days.

The above illustrations of hormonal correlates of fertility indicate that when the estrogen values begin to rise, it signals approaching ovulation with an average warning period of 6 days, and when progesterone rises it signals that ovulation has occurred.

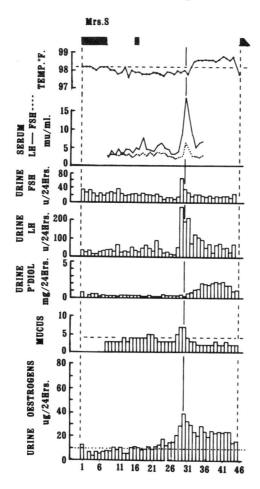

Figure 2–13. The relation between urinary estrogen, pregnanediol, LH and FSH values, serum and FSH, mucous symptoms and basal temperature in a normal cycle. (Brown, 1978)

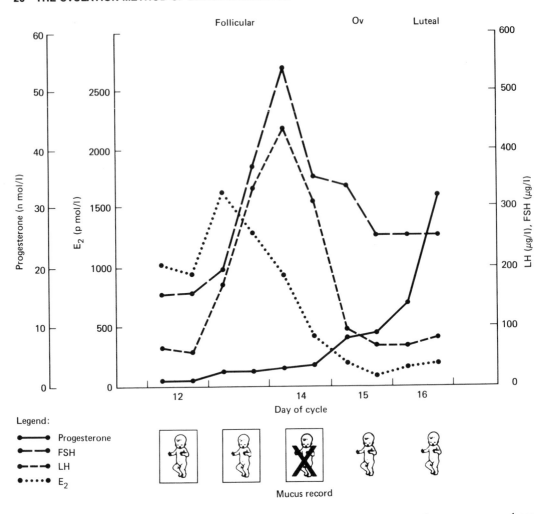

Figure 2–14. Serum estradiol, progesterone, LH, FSH and mucous symptoms in one woman whose day of peak symptom preceded the day of ovulation. The follicular phase has been arbitrarily considered to conclude with the day during which the LH level reaches its peak. The luteal phase has been considered to commence on the day in which the progesterone level exceeds 10 μmol/1. LH and FSH are measured in ug/1 of the L ER 907 pituitary standard. (Casey, 1977)

These ovarian events are controlled by the levels of FSH and LH secreted by the pituitary gland and are reflected by the observable changes in mucous secretions.

In considering all the hormone markers of ovulation available, namely serum and urine LH and FSH, urine estrogens and pregnanediol and plasma estradiol and progesterone, Brown (1978) concluded that any one of these hormone tests, including the peak of LH in serum, could be in error by at least ±1 day and that compared with this, most women could be just as accurate in determining the day of ovulation by their self-observed mucous symptoms. Furthermore, in this study he made a statistical comparison between the onset of fertile mucus and the first rise in estrogen values preceding the estrogen peak; the correlation coefficient between the onset of the two phenomena was 0.91, which was highly significant. Additionally, in 778 observations made by 42 lactating women of mucous symptoms rated on a scale of – 1 (dry) to +9 (fertile), the correlation between the level of urinary estrogen measured at the same time and the mucous symptoms was 0.71, which was also highly significant. Discussion of the statistical reliability of the use-effectiveness of the Ovulation Method is considered in detail in Chapter 11.

Summary

It is clear that the cyclic changes occurring throughout a woman's fertile period of life are under the influence of hormones secreted by the brain, pituitary and ovaries. The ovarian hormones produce identifiable changes in cervical mucous secretions which a woman can learn to recognize. The most important requirement for the self-recognition of the day of ovulation is the identification of the last day of fertile type mucous secretion (the Peak day); most women find this identification to be relatively

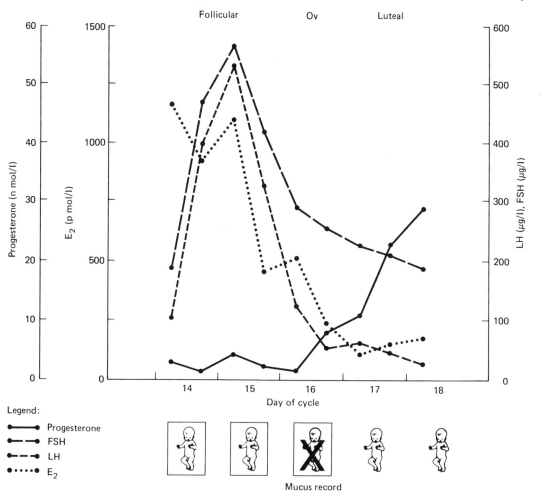

Figure 2–15. Hormonal responses in one woman in whom the day of Peak symptom coincided with the day of ovulation. The follicular and luteal phases have been defined in the legend of Figure 2–14. (Casey 1977)

easy. It has been demonstrated that self-observed changes in mucus from the preovulatory to postovulatory stages of the cycle closely reflect the underlying hormonal events determining fertility. This conclusion is based on comparison of mucous symptoms with urinary and plasma analyses of estrogens, progesterone, LH and FSH, which are scientifically accepted methods of determining ovarian activity and of timing ovulation.

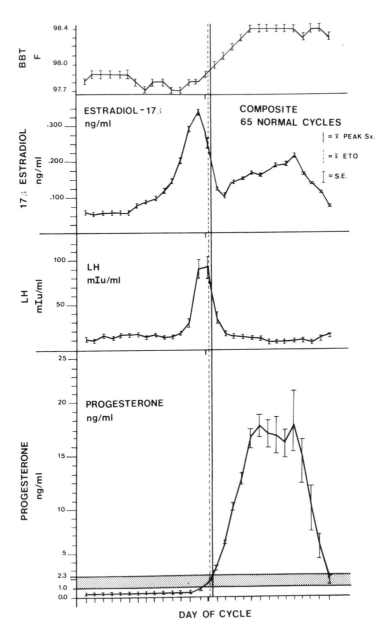

Figure 2–16. The mean serum progesterone, LH, estradiol and basal body temperature (BBT) values for 65 ovulatory cycles showing the estimated time of ovulation (ETO) as the vertical interrupted line and the peak symptom (Peak Sx) as the vertical solid line. The horizontal hatched bar refers to the periovulatory range of progesterone. (Hilgers, T.W., Abraham, G.E. and Cavanaugh, D., 1978).

REFERENCES

Billings, E.L., Billings, J.J., Brown, J.B., and Burger, H. "Symptoms and Hormonal Changes Accompanying Ovulation." *Lancet,* 1972, 282–284.

Brown, J.B. "Urinary Excretion of Estrogens During Pregnancy, Lactation, and the Re-establishment of Menstruation." *Lancet,* 1956, **1,** 704.

Brown, J.B. "Hormonal Correlations of the Ovulation Method." Paper presented at the International Conference on the Ovulation Method, Melbourne, Australia, 1978.

Brown, J.B. and Matthew, G.D. "The Application of Urinary Estrogen Measurements to Problems in Gynecology." *Recent Progress in Hormone Research,* 1962, **18,** 337.

Casey, John H. "Midcycle Hormonal Profiles, Cervical Mucus and Ovulation;" (Abstract). Mott Center Symposium, Wayne State University, Human Ovulation, April, 1977.

Flynn, A.M. and Lynch, S.S. "Cervical Mucus and Indentification of the Fertile Phase of the Menstrual Cycle." *British Journal of Obstetrics and Gynecology,* 1976, **83,** 656–659.

Hilgers, Thomas W., Abraham, Guy E., and Cavanaugh, Denis "Natural Family Planning—I. The Peak Symptom and Estimated Time of Ovulation." *Obstetrics and Gynecology,* November, 1978

3

Observations on Cervical Mucus: Relationship of Mucus to Fertility; Rules for Intercourse

As discussed in Chapter 2, at a certain point in the preovulatory phase of the menstrual cycle, the glands of the cervix produce and secrete a particular kind of mucus that changes markedly in the hours immediately before ovulation. The Ovulation Method of natural family planning is based on the fact that women of all ages, cultures, and educational backgrounds can learn to observe and interpret those changes, and use the information to determine the number and spacing of their children. A couple that wishes to avoid pregnancy abstains from intercourse when the mucus indicates that conception might occur, whereas a couple that wishes to achieve pregnancy has intercourse when the mucus indicates that conception is most likely to occur.

Chapter 3 discusses the types of mucus that can occur during the menstrual cycle and the significance of each type in regard to fertility and intercourse. For clarity and simplicity, the subject is first presented through a discussion of photographs of the mucous secretions at various phases of the ovulatory phase of the cycle.

Throughout the day the mucous secretion (or its absence) can be observed when the vulva is wiped with a tissue after urination. No internal examination is necessary as the latest findings reflect that the woman's observations of the mucus at the opening of the vagina correlate very well with the events that occur at the level of the endocervix (Hilgers and Prebil, 1979).

Consistency, color, and any sensation of wetness or lubrication are the items to be observed.

Figures 3–1 to 3–14 are photographs of the different types of mucous secretion of one woman during one menstrual cycle. When studying the photographs, the reader should remember that what is shown is the mucous pattern of one woman, not of every woman. The amount of mucus and the number of days each type of mucus is secreted varies from cycle to cycle in the same woman. Nevertheless, the photographs are useful since the pattern is similar among all women.

Figure 3–1 shows the mucus as it first appeared. The secretion was slight, creamy, cloudy, and not elastic. That first secretion alerted the woman to the fact that ovulation was likely to occur in a matter of days.

The mucous secretion can begin as early as the first days of menstruation, but in special circumstances (breast-feeding, for example) it may not begin for months (see pages 81, 83, 84 and 85). In the woman discussed in these photographs, the mucous secretion began at different times in nearly every cycle–a variation that is perfectly normal. For the cycle shown, mucus began 4 days after menstruation commenced.

Figure 3–2 shows the mucous secretion on the second day. The secretion was sticky, creamy, and inelastic. It was still cloudy. When the mucus of the second day was stretched more than an inch or so, it broke (Figure 3–3).

Figure 3–4 shows the mucus as it appeared on the third day. It was still creamy. Note that there was more mucus on the third than on the first and second days. Many, but not all, women experience such an increase in quantity, but it is the quality of the mucus that is important, not its quantity. When the mucus was held between the fingers of one hand (Figure 3–5), it was shown to be more elastic than it was on the first and second days. It was still creamy and cloudy, but it was more watery and somewhat lumpy.

By the evening of the third day, the mucus had changed markedly (Figure 3–6). It had become almost clear, resembling the white of a raw egg. The change was a most important one since it signaled the onset of the period of greatest fertility.

By the morning of the fourth day of secretion, the mucus had increased in quantity while remaining clear (Figure 3–7). The mucus of the fourth day could be stretched several inches without its breaking (Figure 3–8). Elasticity is a most significant characteristic of fertile mucus, as explained on page 7. Figure 3–9 further illustrates the clearness and elasticity of the mucus of the fourth day.

By 2 p.m. of the fourth day, the mucous secretion had become yellow-brown, opaque, and sticky (Figure 3–10. The change from the clear, elastic mucus of that morning indicated that ovulation had occurred or would occur within a few hours (Brown, 1978, Casey, 1978).

As shown in Figure 3–11, the mucus on the morning of the fifth day was a sticky, cloudy gel, with some traces of clear mucus *(top, right)*. The rise in progesterone after ovulation makes the mucus acquire this characteristic change.

On the sixth day, the gel-type mucus diminished in quantity (Figure 3–12).

On the seventh day, a thick, cloudy, milky mucus was present, and in smaller quantity (Figure 3–13).

On the eighth day, there was no observable mucous secretion (Figure 3–14). Such a day is referred to as a dry day. The woman under discussion had dry days until the end of the cycle.

RELATIONSHIP OF MUCUS TO FERTILITY

The mucus secreted by the glands of the cervix is related to fertility in the following ways.

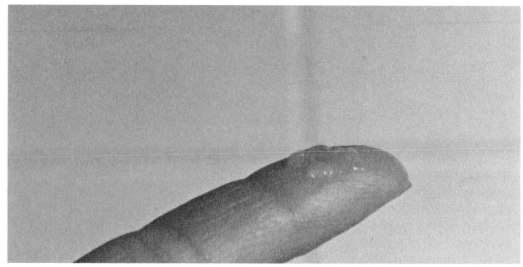

Figure 3–1. The mucus as it first appeared.

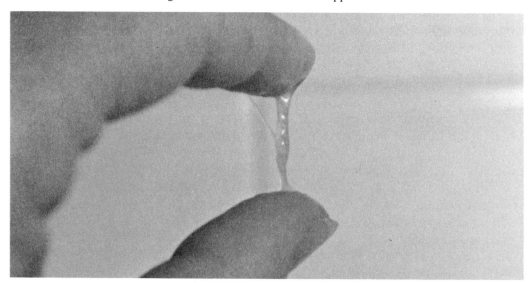

Figure 3–2. The mucus as it appeared on the second day.

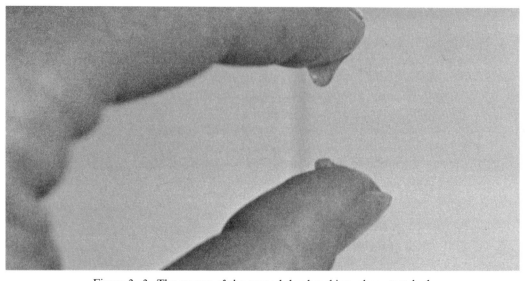

Figure 3–3. The mucus of the second day breaking when stretched.

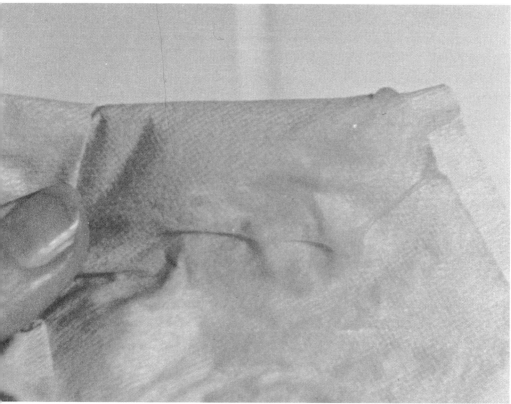

Figure 3–4. The mucus as observed in tissue paper on the third day.

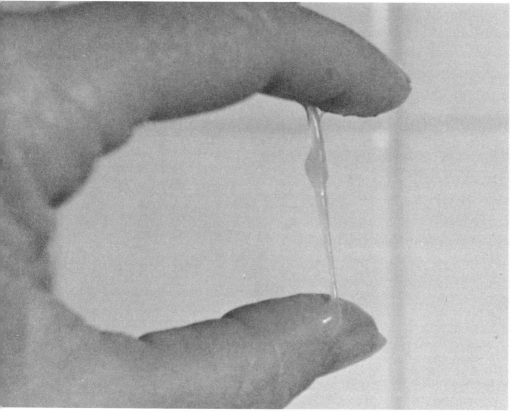

Figure 3–5. The mucus collected from tissue paper showing increased stretchability on the third day.

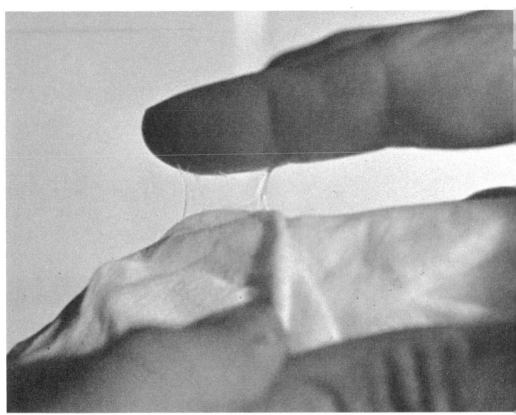
Figure 3-6. The mucus as it changed by the evening of the third day.

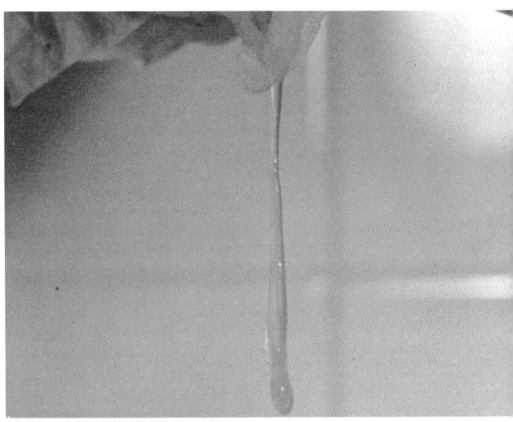
Figure 3-7. The mucus as it appeared on the morning of the fourth day.

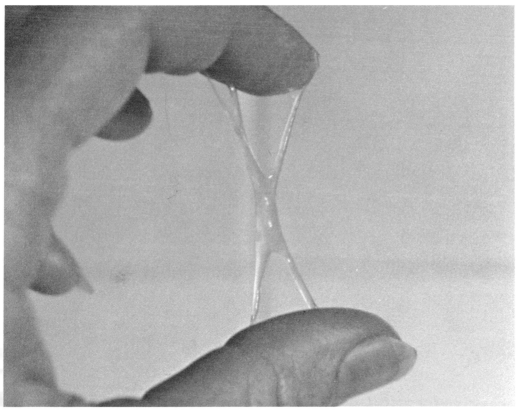

Figure 3–8. The mucus showing its transparency on the morning of the fourth day.

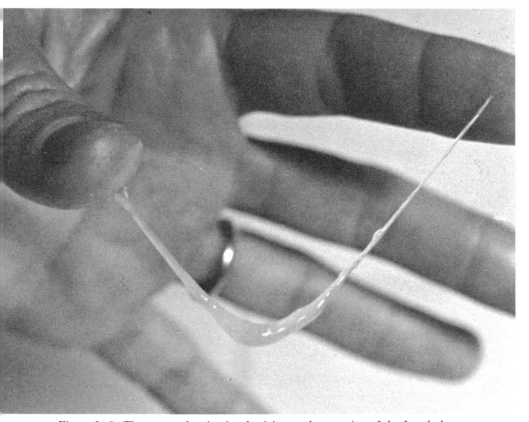

Figure 3–9. The mucus showing its elasticity on the morning of the fourth day.

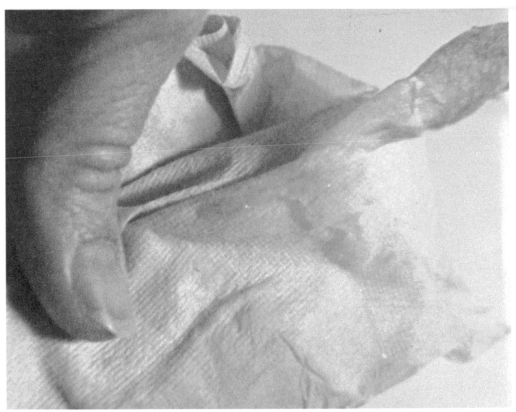

Figure 3–10. The mucus as it appeared on the afternoon of the fourth day.

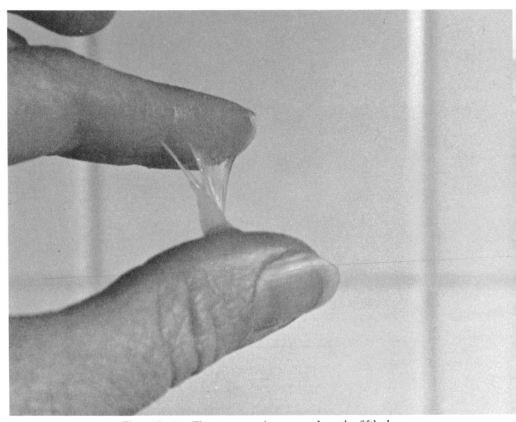

Figure 3–11. The mucus as it appeared on the fifth day.

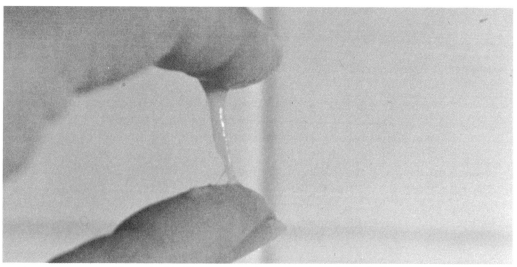

Figure 3–12. The mucus as it appeared on the sixth day.

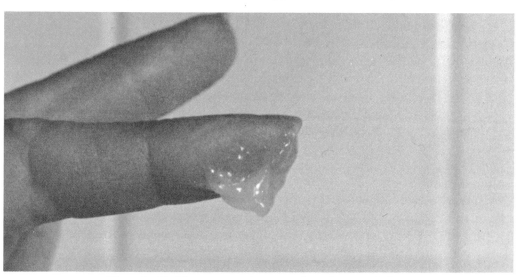

Figure 3–13. The mucus as it appeared on the seventh day.

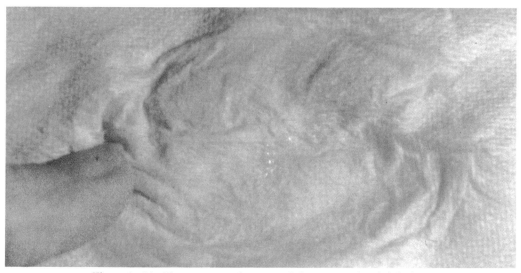

Figure 3–14. The return to almost total dryness on the eighth day.

1. It provides lubrication for intercourse.

2. Sticky, cloudy mucus (often referred to as infertile mucus) impedes the sperm's transport toward the ovum, whereas clear, elastic mucus (often referred to as fertile mucus) favors the transport of the sperm. (See also pages 26 through 31.)

3. Clear, elastic mucus protects the sperm from the acid environment of the vagina.

4. Clear, elastic mucus provides some of the sperm's energy requirements.

5. It has been theorized that clear, elastic mucus may help "capacitate" the sperm cells. Capacitation is the process by which a sperm becomes able to fertilize an ovum. It is believed sperm must be in the woman's body for some hours before it is capable of penetrating and thus fertilizing the ovum.

OVULATION

Although ovulation was discussed in detail in Chapter 2, a few comments on the process are pertinent here.

Ovulation can occur on only one day in the cycle. If pregnancy does not occur in a particular cycle, menstruation follows about two weeks after ovulation. The timespan between ovulation and the following menstrual period varies from 11 to 16 days. The time from the beginning of the cycle up to ovulation, however, can vary quite a bit—ovulation can occur during the menstrual period itself (page 51), or it may not occur until weeks, even months, after a menstrual period has ended (Pages 55 and 56). Thus a cycle can be long or short, its duration depending on when ovulation occurs. The length of the cycle varies from woman to woman, and from month to month in the same woman.

Contrary to a popular belief, a woman cannot ovulate several times a month at widely spaced intervals. If more than one ovum is released (as happens in the case of fraternal twins), the evidence seems to indicate that the second ovum is released simultaneously with the first one (Brown, 1977). Certain factors can *delay* ovulation, as explained on page 71, but an ovulation that can result in pregnancy is usually preceded by the warning mucus signs (pages 26 through 31).

Changes That Signal the Imminence of Ovulation

The following changes in the mucous secretion indicate that ovulation will take place in a matter of hours.

1. The mucus changes in consistency—from sticky, cloudy mucus (Figure 3–1) to clear, elastic mucus (Figure 3–8).

2. The woman feels a lubricating or a wet sensation in the vulva. The sensation is caused by the change in the water content of the mucus. (Mucus is about 92 percent water in the first days of its appearance; as ovulation draws close, the water content of the mucus increases to about 98 percent.) The lubricating sensation may last for one or more days, and it is obvious to the woman as she goes about her daily activities.

The lubricating sensation and the elasticity are more reliable signs of ovulation in those instances when the mucus secreted right before ovulation is tinged with blood and has a brownish, cloudy appearance (page 59).

The last day of clear, elastic mucus is referred to as the Peak day, so called because that day is thought to be the day of peak fertility, as well as the time most closely related to peak levels of the ovarian hormones (page 5). The Peak day can be recognized as such only in retrospect—from the woman's observation on the following day of either dryness or of the return of sticky, cloudy mucus. Accuracy in detecting the Peak day can be determined by relating the Peak day to the first day of the following menstrual period, which normally occurs about two weeks later.

RULES FOR INTERCOURSE WHEN PREGNANCY IS TO BE AVOIDED

It must be understood that the rules apply not only to intercourse but to every other kind of contact between the sexual organs, including coitus interruptus, intercourse protected by contraceptives of any kind, and even *simple genital contact.* Sexual arousal in the man—even if he doesn't ejaculate—can produce secretions that may contain sperm which can be transported by the fertile mucus outside the vagina, thus conception can occur.

Early Day Rules For the Pre-ovulatory Phase

1. *Intercourse should not take place* during menstruation or on any other days of bleeding. Since the mucous secretion could begin during (and be masked by) menstruation, it is possible that ovulation could occur during menstruation or immediately after it (Figure 5-3 A, B, C, D, E).

2. *Intercourse can take place* from the end of the menstrual period until the first day of the sticky, cloudy mucous secretion. The days from the end of the menstrual period until the beginning of the sticky, cloudy mucus are normally dry days. They are sometimes referred to as the early safe days.

Until the woman has experience in distinguishing seminal fluid from mucus,[1] it is safer to avoid intercourse on the day *following* intercourse and to restrict it to the evenings.

In some long cycles, there may be a succession of three or more days on which mucus is present. The mucus may stop for a number of days, then begin again. Until the woman has become experienced in distinguishing fertile and infertile mucus, it is safer to avoid intercourse on any day when mucus is present, and until the evening of the fourth day after these "patches" of mucus disappear, as she is still in the preovulatory phase of her cycle and the early day rules apply.

[1] Seminal fluid foams—and may even stretch a bit—when rolled between the fingers, but it quickly breaks and disappears as water would.

Rules for the Post Ovulatory Phase

1. *Intercourse should not take place* from the first appearance of mucus until the fourth day after the Peak day. (The Peak day is counted as zero.) The rule is sometimes called the Peak rule. Although the sticky, cloudy mucus that first appears is considered to have contraceptive properties (see page 32), the abstinence rule allows for any human error in the woman's observation of the actual time of the first appearance of the mucus. If the woman has not accurately noted the first appearance of the mucus her estimate of when ovulation would occur would be thrown off, and pregnancy might result if she had intercourse too close to ovulation.

The Peak rule takes into account the close time-relationship of the Peak day to ovulation—it allows time for ovulation to occur and for the ovum to die.

2. *Intercourse can take place* from the fourth day after the Peak until the first day of the following menstrual period. Whether the woman has dry days or an infertile mucous secretion (page 75) the rule holds, because the ovum which lives only about 12 hours after ovulation, has disintegrated and the woman is infertile.

3. *Intercourse should not take place* on any day of bleeding between menstrual periods nor until the fourth day after the cessation of such bleeding.

4. If there should be any recurrence of mucus in the days between the Peak day and the next menstrual period, the characteristics of the mucus should be noted. If the mucus is elastic or if it produces a lubricating sensation, intercourse may not take place any day mucus is present and until the fourth day.

For simplicity, the rules for intercourse given here cover only the usual circumstances. The rules concerning intercourse during special circumstances, such as lactation, menopause, mucus patches, and continuous mucus discharge, are given in Chapters 7 and 8, at the point where the particular topic is discussed.

The rules for intercourse that apply when the couple wishes to have a child are given in Chapter 6.

REFERENCES

Brown, J.B. 1977. Personal communication.

Brown, J.B. "Hormonal Correlations of the Ovulation Method." Paper presented at the International Conference on the Ovulation Method, Melbourne, Australia, 1978.

Casey, John H. "Midcycle Hormonal Profiles, Cervical Mucus and Ovulation," (Abstract). Mott Center Symposium, Wayne State University, Human Ovulation, April, 1977.

Hilgers, Thomas W., Abraham, Guy E., and Cavanagh, Denis. "Natural Family Planning—I. The Peak Symptom and Estimated Time of Ovulation." *Obstetrics and Gynecology,* November, 1978.

Hilgers, Thomas W. and Prebil, Ann M. The Ovulation Method-Vulvar Observations as an Index of Fertility/Infertility, *"Obstetrics and Gynecology,"* 12:22, 1979.

4

Charting Information About the Menstrual Cycle

Chapter 4 gives directions for charting the observations the woman makes on her mucous secretions and on other aspects of her menstrual cycle.

In 1970 a simple chart was devised to be used by people in illiterate communities. The chart proved so effective that it is now used by people of all levels of education throughout the world. As shown in Figure 4–1, the chart is made up of blocks on which the woman is to paste a particular kind of stamp at the end of each day to signify what she has observed about her menstrual cycle that day.

It is strongly recommended that a woman who is beginning to learn the Ovulation Method abstain from intercourse for an entire cycle so that she can observe the normal pattern of the cycle. This way she is given a chance to learn and observe her normal pattern of fertility and infertility without the fear of pregnancy on her first learning cycle.

Three kinds of stamps are in general use—red stamps, green stamps, and white baby stamps (Figure 4–1).

The red stamps are used to indicate days of menstrual bleeding and any other kind of bleeding from the vagina that is not accompanied by an observable mucous secretion. Couples who wish to avoid pregnancy should not have intercourse on days marked with red stamps since those days are possibly fertile (pages 51 and 52).

The green stamps are used to indicate (1) the dry days between menstruation and ovulation; and (2) all the days from the fourth day after the Peak day until the first day of the following menstrual period. Couples who wish to avoid pregnancy should confine intercourse to days marked with green stamps.

The white baby stamps are used to indicate (1) days between menstruation and ovulation on which there is a mucous secretion; (2) the three days after the Peak day, which are days of possible fertility; (3) days of bleeding on which a mucous secretion is observed; and (4) the day after intercourse, unless the woman has experience in distinguishing seminal fluid from a mucous secretion (page 38).

An X is marked across the appropriate white baby stamp to indicate the Peak day, which, as explained on page 38, can be known only in retrospect.

Since the menstrual cycle is generally considered to start with the menstrual period, the chart should begin with the first day of menstruation. Nevertheless, women are asked to begin charting the day they are instructed regardless what phase of their cycle they may be experiencing and to begin a new line when menstruation begins. The date of the first day of menstruation is written in the left-hand margin, and each evening the appropriate stamp is placed in the block for that day. It is important that the charting be done every day (the woman should not rely on her memory) and at the end of the day (so that all the changes that occurred during the day can be noted).

It is important that information be kept on the various aspects of the menstrual cycle, especially for the woman who is new to the Method. Information about what happened on a particular day can be coded on the stamp itself or written on the block immediately under the stamp, and the charting of the next menstrual cycle can begin on the line under that (Figure 4-2).

Figure 4-2 is a composite photograph whose parts have been assembled to illustrate certain relationships in the menstrual cycle. a) It is a chart of one menstrual cycle. c) It shows the detailed description the woman made of the mucous secretion. b) It shows how sticky, cloudy (viscous) mucus retards the motility of the sperm and that clear, elastic (less viscous) mucus helps sperm motility. d) It shows how much mucus might be present. (The quantity can vary from woman to woman and from cycle to cycle in the same woman.) The quantity of the mucus is not as significant as are its other characteristics, as explained on page 25. Figure 4-2 also shows the changes in mucus at various points in the cycle—from (1) sticky, cloudy mucus at the beginning of the secretion to (2) clear, elastic mucus when ovulation is very close; (3) sticky, cloudy mucus after ovulation. The changes in the mucus reflect the changes in the levels of estrogen and progesterone.

It is possible to keep a record of the menstrual cycles of an entire year on one sheet of paper (Figure 4-1), readily available for analysis by the woman herself, or by her teacher in the Ovulation Method, or by her physician.

Figure 4-3 shows an 8-year record of a 38-year-old woman. Her cycles show a great deal of regularity, broken only in the very first cycle, when ovulation was delayed. The woman in question remarked that the time of that cycle was one of great pressure that subsided shortly before the onset of ovulation. The observation confirms the finding that stress can result in a delay in ovulation (pages 67 and 68).

Note in Figure 4-3 that in the last three years of charting, the woman used yellow stamps. Yellow stamps were introduced in 1974 to help women distinguish fertile mucus from infertile mucus. The yellow stamps may be used in the following circumstances.

Figure 4-1. A chart showing red, green, and white stamps in position. This type of chart, originally devised for people in illiterate communities, proved so effective that it is now used by people of all levels of education.

Figure 4-2. a. A record of one menstrual cycle. b. The effect of the mucous secretion on sperm motility. c. A description of the mucous secretion. d. Characteristics of mucus.

Figure 4-3. An eight-year-record. The cycles are consistently regular in the post-ovulatory phase.

Figure 4-4. The Ovulation Wheel, a device that summarizes information about the fertility of the various phases of the cycle.

Figure 4-5. A woman's basic infertile pattern can be either dry days or days of continuous infertile mucous secretion.

Fig. 4-1

Typical One Year Record. Normal Cycles
United States

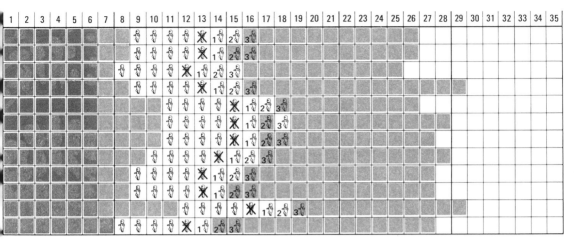

NOTE: **I** = Intercourse

Fig. 4-4

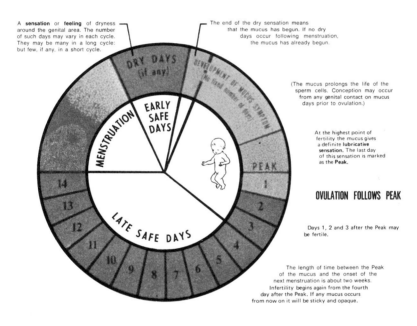

A **sensation** or **feeling** of dryness around the genital area. The number of such days may vary in each cycle. They may be many in a long cycle; but few, if any, in a short cycle.

The end of the dry sensation means that the mucus has begun. If no dry days occur following menstruation, the mucus has already begun.

(The mucus prolongs the life of the sperm cells. Conception may occur from any genital contact on mucus days prior to ovulation.)

At the highest point of fertility the mucus gives a definite **lubricative sensation.** The last day of this sensation is marked as the **Peak.**

OVULATION FOLLOWS PEAK

Days 1, 2 and 3 after the Peak may be fertile.

The length of time between the Peak of the mucus and the onset of the next menstruation is about two weeks. Infertility begins again from the fourth day after the Peak. If any mucus occurs from now on it will be sticky and opaque.

Fig. 4-5

1	2	3	4	5	6	7	8	9	10	11	12	13	14	15	16	17	18	19	20	21	22	23	24	25	26	27	28	29	30	31	32	33	34	35

OVULATION METHOD
Figure 4-2

Normal Cycles

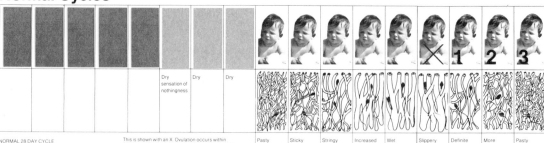

| | | | | Dry sensation of nothingness | Dry | Dry | | | | | | | | | |

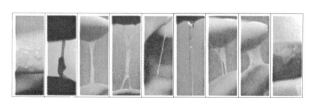

NORMAL 28 DAY CYCLE
This cycle shows 5 days of menstrual bleeding indicated with red stamps followed by 3 plain green stamps to record days when there is a sensation of dryness known as the Basic Infertile Pattern. The dry (plain green) days are safe days (infertile) unless preceded by mucus. White stamps with the imprint of a baby are used when the first day of mucus secretion is observed in the tissue paper. Those wishing to postpone pregnancy must abstain from intercourse from this day on until 3 days after peak or day of ovulation. As ovulation approaches the mucus changes, it usually becomes clearer and stretches without breaking like the raw white of an egg. the amount may increase or decrease and is sometimes tinged with blood. The last day of the slippery lubricative mucus is the "peak symptom."

This is shown with an X. Ovulation occurs within 24 hours of the peak. Abstention is required for the 3 days following the peak symptom. After the peak, a **definite change** is observed, there is no longer a feeling of wetness and the mucus has become opaque and sticky (white baby stamp) or a sensation of dryness is observed (green baby stamp). White stamps with the imprint of a baby are used if sticky opaque mucus is present, and green baby stamps if the mucus has stopped and there is a sensation of dryness.
Infertility returns on the fourth day following the peak giving freedom for intercourse to those who wish to avoid pregnancy.
For those wishing to achieve pregnancy, intercourse is recommended on the days when clear stretchy mucus is observed.

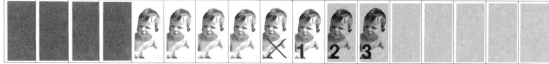

| Pasty not elastic breaks if stretched | Sticky opaque a little stretchy | Stringy more elastic | Increased elasticity clearer slight wet sensation | Wet sensation more watery transparent | Slippery slimy sensation very clear like raw egg white | Definite change sticky cloudy pasty yellow tinge | More sticky milky looking tacky | Pasty sticky |

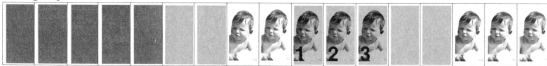

Short Cycles

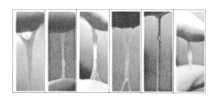

SHORT CYCLE
It is possible for the process of ovulation to begin before the menstrual period has ended as shown above. The mucus secretion occurs early in this cycle making it possible for the days of bleeding to obscure the beginning of the fertile pattern. For this reason, it is necessary to avoid intercourse during menstruation if pregnancy is not desired.

Long Cycles

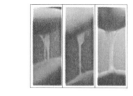

LONG CYCLE
Long cycles may have many dry days (Basic Infertile Pattern) or as shown above, the dry days may be interrupted by patches of mucus. Intercourse should be avoided for 3 days following any secretion until after ovulation has occured. The pattern of fertility simply occurs later in a long cycle with menstruation following 12 to 16 days after the peak symptom, exactly as it does in a short or normal cycle.

Intermittent patches of mucus in the pre-ovulatory phase often occur in nursing mothers, premenopausal women and particularly those coming off the pill.

CODE FOR STAMPS:

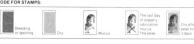

| Bleeding or spotting | Dry | Mucus | The last day of slippery lubricative mucus. The peak | Dry after peak for 3 days |

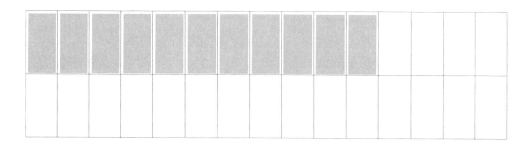

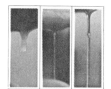

Figure 4-3

TYPICAL EIGHT YEAR RECORD. NORMAL CYCLES

NOTE: **I** = Intercourse

Figure 4-3 (continued)

TYPICAL EIGHT YEAR RECORD. NORMAL CYCLES
UNITED STATES

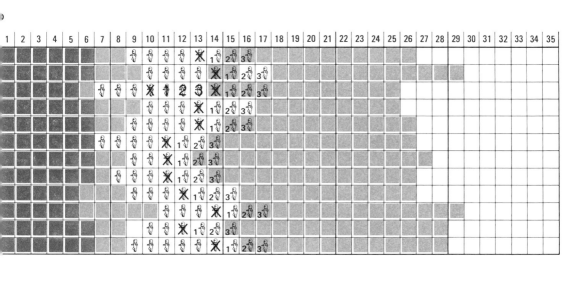

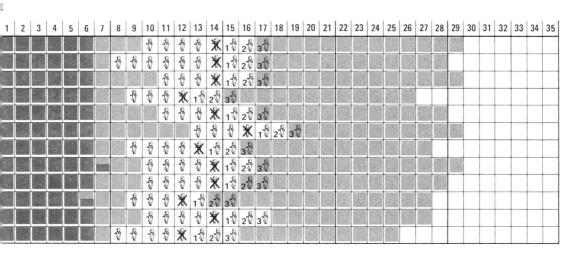

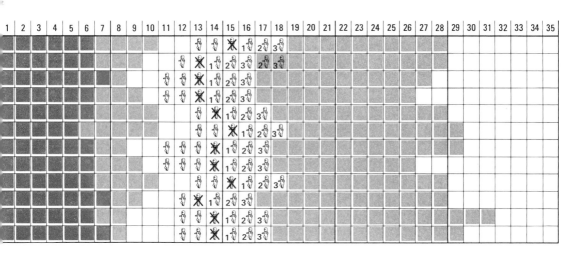

G.

H.

NOTE: **I** = Intercourse

1. In the luteal phase of the cycle to record any mucus that occurs from the fourth day after the Peak day until the beginning of the next menstrual cycle.

2. To record the continuous mucous discharge that can be a woman's basic infertile pattern. A woman's basic infertile mucous secretion—mucus that does not show any changes in amount, color, or any other characteristics—Figure 4–5 shows how both types of basic infertile pattern are recorded (see Figure 4–5, page 37).

Carefully kept charts are fascinating documents that help a woman—and her doctor—learn more about her body, and enable her to take control of her own reproductive life.

Summary

The graphic device shown in Figure 4–2 is an excellent summary of the information presented in Chapters 3 and 4.

REFERENCE

Billings, E.L., Billings, J.J., and Catarinich, M., *Atlas of the Ovulation Method,* Third Edition. Melbourne, Australia: Advocate Press, May, 1977.

5

Charts of Normal, Irregular, and Anovulatory Cycles

Chapter 5 discusses normal cycles, irregular cycles, and cycles that are possibly anovulatory. Charts from women all over the world are used to illustrate that (1) the characteristics of the mucous secretions are common to women of all countries and cultures; and (2) women everywhere are able to accurately record their observations of the mucous secretions and thus either achieve pregnancy or avoid it.

CHARTING NORMAL CYCLES

The charts of women from the United States, Gilbert and Ellice Islands, India, Puerto Rico, Guatemala, and Nigeria (Figure 5–1) show that the ovulatory phase of the menstrual cycle (white baby stamps) appeared regularly. As expected, the length of the luteal phase (that is, from ovulation to menstruation) was relatively constant—11 to 16 days—whereas the length of the follicular phase (that is, from menstruation to ovulation) was more varied.

In addition to the stamps described in Chapter 4, the women whose charts are shown in Figure 5–1 used yellow baby stamps, and green baby stamps. The yellow baby stamps were used to indicate any cloudy, sticky mucus in the three days after the Peak day. If there was no secretion in the three days after the Peak day, green baby stamps were used to indicate dryness but possible fertility. As explained in Chapter 4, the yellow stamps were used to indicate cloudy, sticky mucus.

Occasionally, a cloudy, sticky secretion occurs in the middle of the luteal phase (Figure 5–1C). When such is the case—and if pregnancy is to be avoided—the following rule for intercourse should be observed:

If the woman has even one day of fertile mucus, she must abstain that day and for the three following days. That rule holds for both preovulatory and the postovulatory

Figure 5–1. The ovulatory phase of the cycle appeared regularly. Note the variations in length of the follicular phase. The luteal phase was relatively constant.

Figure 5–2. Even women who cannot read or write are able to keep accurate charts and apply the rules of the Ovulation Method.

Normal Cycles
Women Were Literate

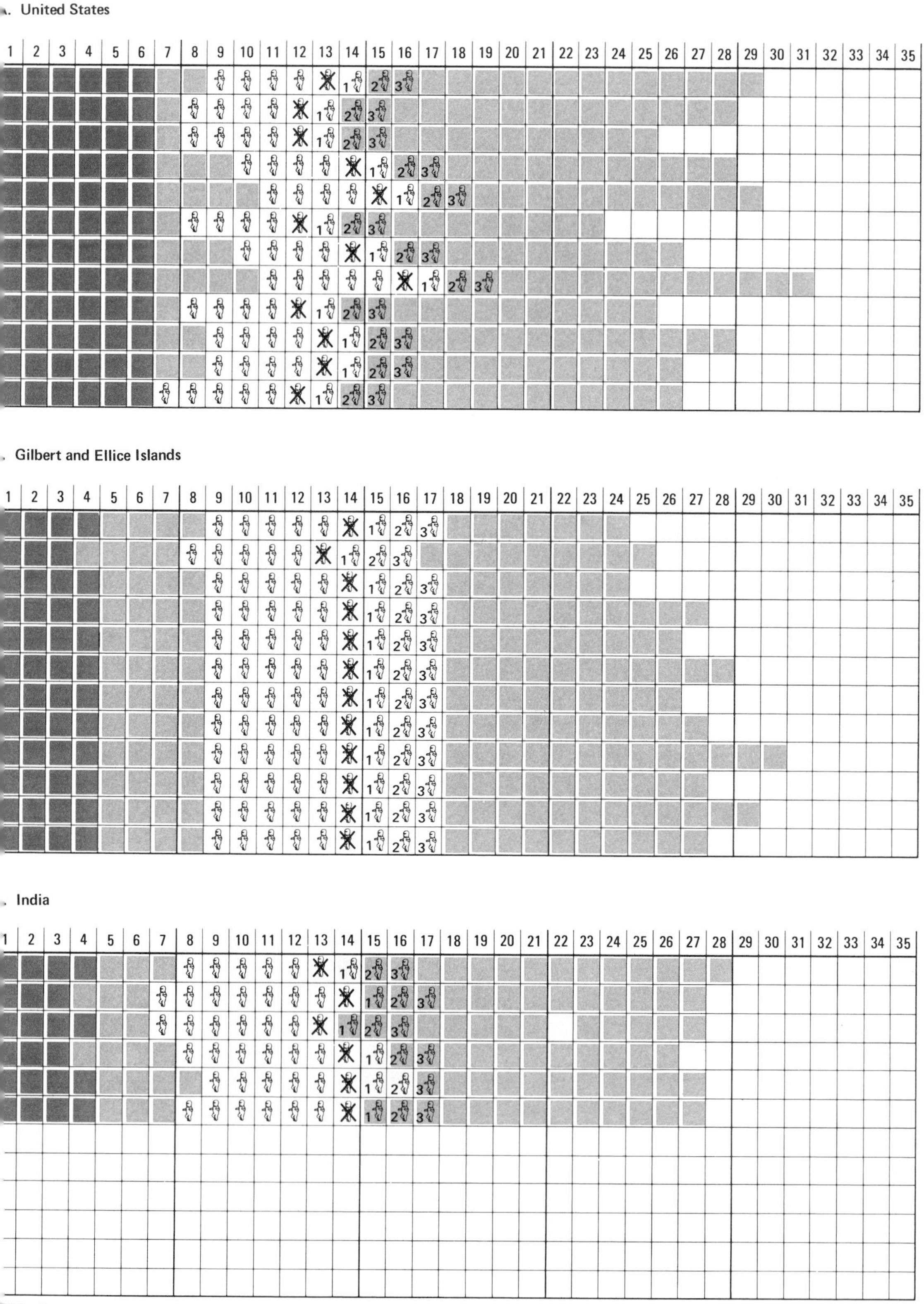

A. United States

B. Gilbert and Ellice Islands

C. India

NOTE: **I** = Intercourse

Figure 5-1 (continued)

Normal Cycles (continued)
Women Were Literate

D. Puerto Rico

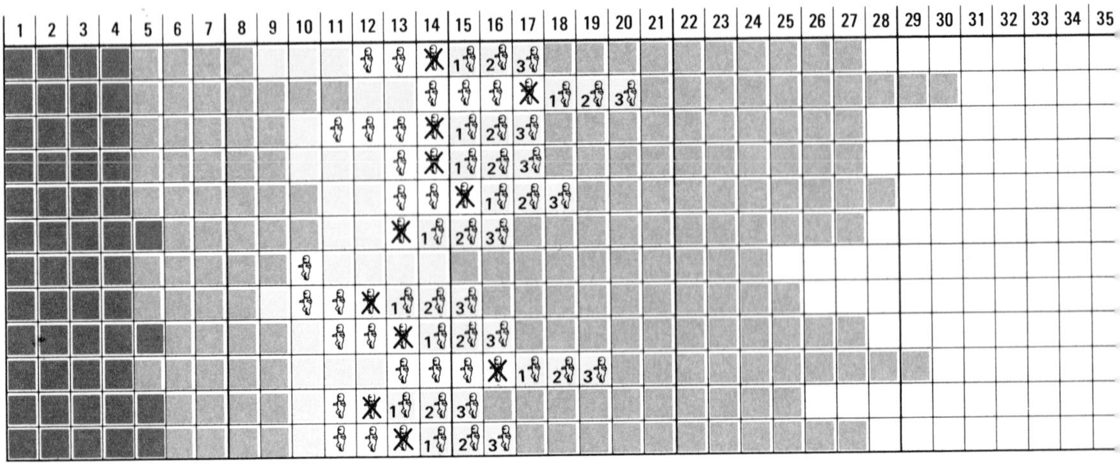

E. Guatemala

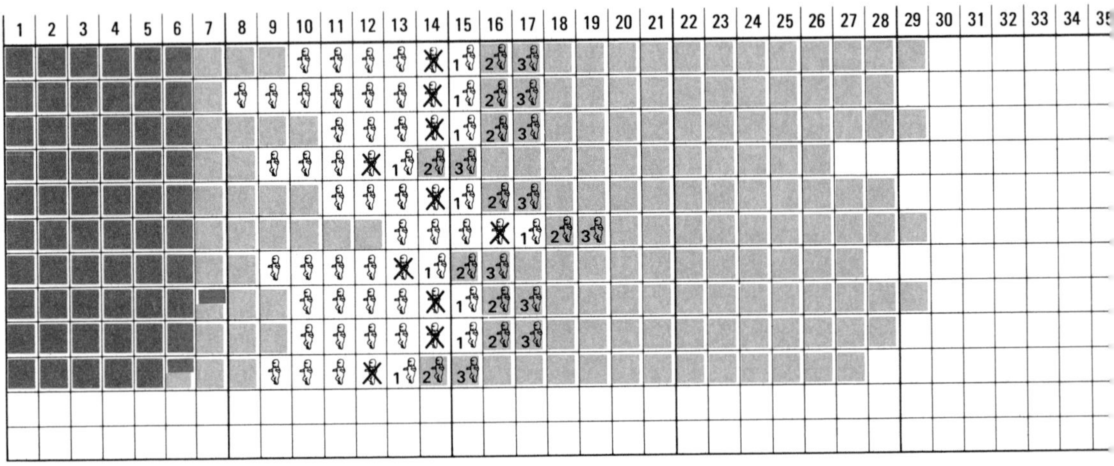

F. Nigeria

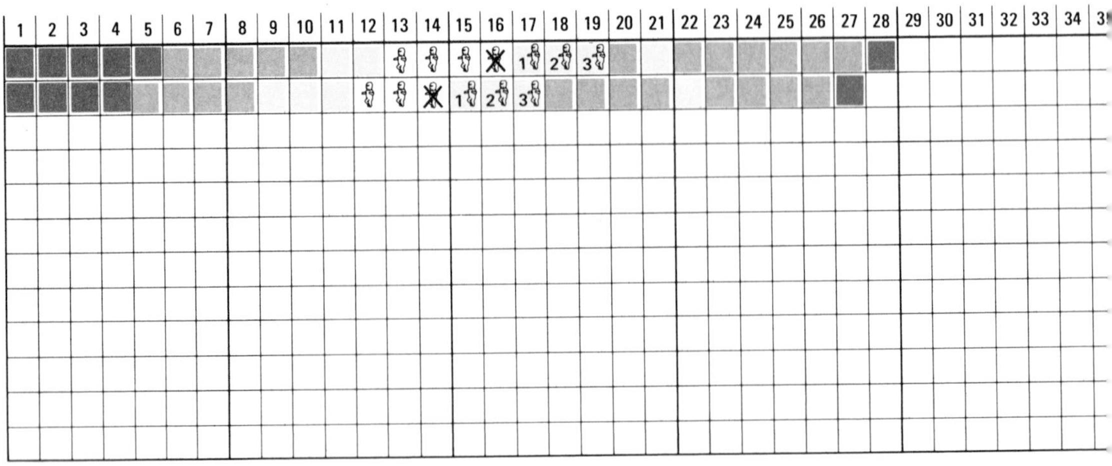

NOTE: **I** = Intercourse

Normal Cycles
Women were Illiterate

Guatemala
18 Month Record

| 1 | 2 | 3 | 4 | 5 | 6 | 7 | 8 | 9 | 10 | 11 | 12 | 13 | 14 | 15 | 16 | 17 | 18 | 19 | 20 | 21 | 22 | 23 | 24 | 25 | 26 | 27 | 28 | 29 | 30 | 31 | 32 | 33 | 34 | 35 |

Nigeria

| 2 | 3 | 4 | 5 | 6 | 7 | 8 | 9 | 10 | 11 | 12 | 13 | 14 | 15 | 16 | 17 | 18 | 19 | 20 | 21 | 22 | 23 | 24 | 25 | 26 | 27 | 28 | 29 | 30 | 31 | 32 | 33 | 34 | 35 |

E: **I** = Intercourse

Figure 5-2 (continued)

Normal Cycles (continued)
Women were Illiterate

C. Korea

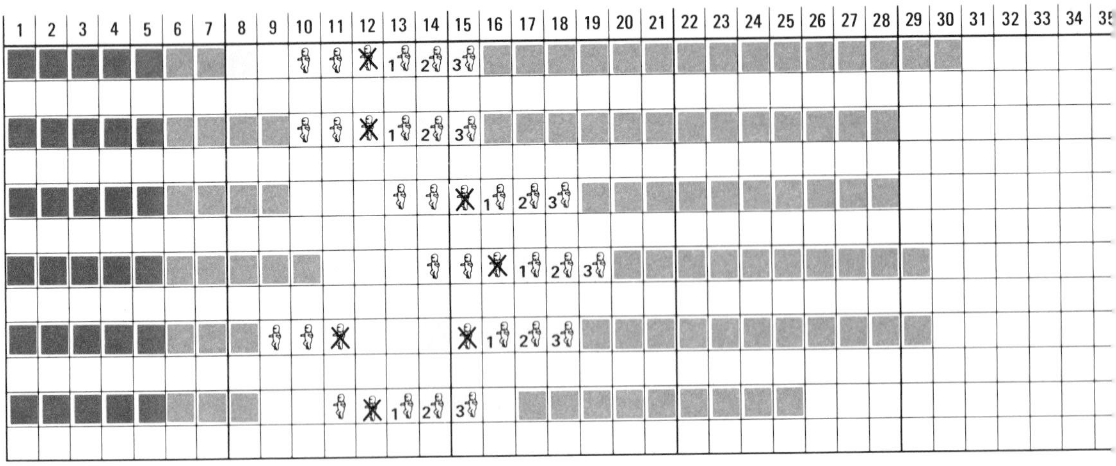

D. Fiji

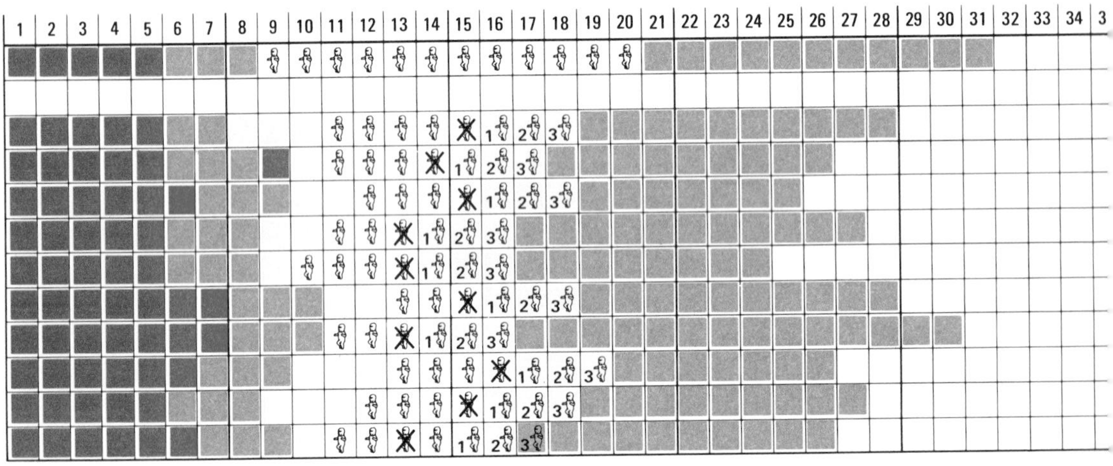

E. Papua New Guinea

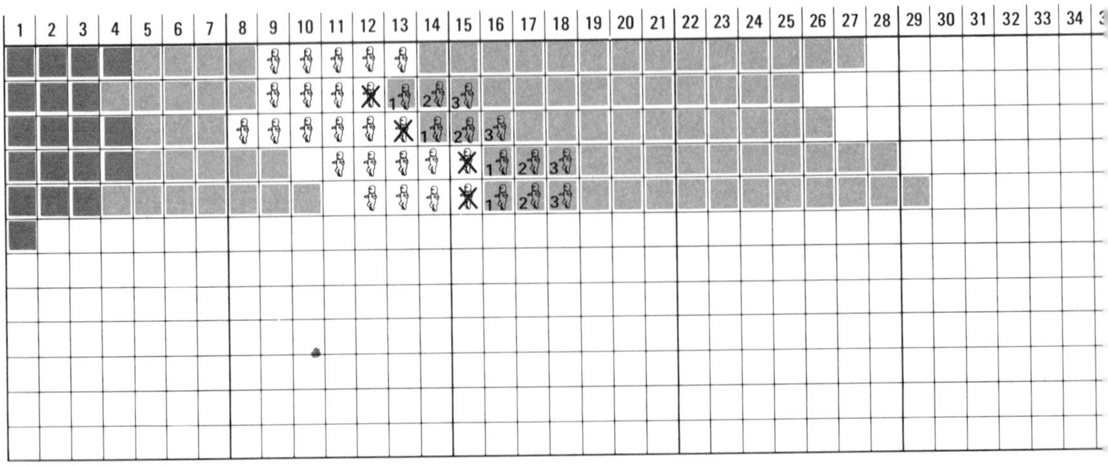

NOTE: I = Intercourse

phases of the cycle. After the woman gains experience in distinguishing fertile mucus from infertile mucus the following rules apply:

1. If one or two days of cloudy, sticky mucus are followed by a dry day, *intercourse may take place* safely on the dry day.

2. If three days of cloudy, sticky mucus are present, intercourse may not take place safely during those days and for three days after.

These rules are based on extensive teaching experience (see pages 33 and 34).

Figure 5–2 shows charts of women from Guatemala, Nigeria, Korea, Fiji, and Papua New Guinea. The women could not read or write. (References to illiteracy are made here and in other chapters only to underscore the important fact that women of all levels of education and types of culture, are able to understand and use the Ovulation Method.)

The 18-month record of a woman from Guatemala, of proven fertility, (Figure 5–2A) shows regular cycles of normal length (27 to 33 days).

Figures 5–2B and 5–2E shows the charts of women from Nigeria and Papua New Guinea. The women were 35 and 25 years old, respectively, and they were known to be fertile. They had fewer days of mucous secretion than had the women from the other countries represented in the chart. That phenomenon may be related to the fact that both women were from small villages (in which the diet was probably poor) and thus possibly had nutritional deficiencies.

Figure 5–2C shows the record of a woman from Korea. The cycles were regular until the fifth one. In that cycle the ovulatory phase was interrupted by illness. It resumed after three days (see also Figure 7–2, page 69). Figure 5–2D shows the chart of a woman from Fiji. Women are first taught to place a white baby stamp from the first day mucus is observed. Most women at first are generally overcautious, and thus place a large number of white baby stamps. As they gain experience they learn to distinguish the two types of mucus, which leads fairly early to the use of the yellow stamps.

The teacher of the Ovulation Method in Fiji found it easier to call the types of mucus simply mucus Type 1 (sticky, cloudy mucus) and Type 2 mucus (clear, elastic mucus). Note (Figure 5–2D) that from cycle 2 to the end of the chart, Type 1 mucus (yellow stamps) was followed by Type 2 mucus (white baby stamps) and then by Type 1 mucus (yellow baby stamps). Note also that as the woman gained experience in distinguishing the two types of mucus, the number of days of abstinence was considerably reduced.

CHARTING SHORT CYCLES

The charts in Figure 5–3 are those of women from Canada, the United States, Guatemala, Mexico, and Papua New Guinea who had short cycles. Note that in the majority of the cycles, menstruation and the beginning of the mucous secretion overlapped, as can be inferred from the white baby stamps early in the cycles. Since the mucous secretions begin early in women who have short cycles, abstinence from intercourse during menstruation is mandatory if pregnancy is to be avoided.

Figure 5–3D shows a particularly interesting record. The woman was Mexican, 25 years old, and illiterate. She had married at the age of 15, and she had eight children at the time of her introduction to the Ovulation Method. She told the instructor that they used to restrict intercourse to the menstrual periods because they had thought that the menstrual days were the only infertile ones. To their dismay, she became pregnant time and again. Now, after some experience with charting, this woman realizes that her ovulatory phase and menstruation overlap. She has since been using the Ovulation Method successfully to avoid pregnancy. The white baby stamps at the end of the cycles in Figure 5–3D mark the mucous secretion that is often present just before menstruation. Usually the mucus is a creamy or yellow-brown color right before menstruation (Figure 5–3F). The mucous secretion is probably a result of the disintegration of the lining of the uterus and indicates the beginning of menstruation, whereby the lining is shed and renewed. Some women have a clear, elastic secretion just before bleeding. Such a secretion at that time may indicate that the cycle was anovulatory (Brown, 1978).

CHARTING LONG, IRREGULAR CYCLES

The charts in Figure 5–4 show long, irregular cycles in women from Canada, Korea, and Fiji. Even women with such irregularities are able to recognize their fertile phases because the mucus gives advance notice of ovulation.

Figure 5–4A shows an irregular pattern in a Canadian woman. In the six cycles shown, the woman apparently ovulated only once (cycle 1). The woman's daughter (Figure 5–4B) showed the same irregularity, probably because of hereditary reasons or because the pair may have had similar nutritional deficiencies. Like her mother, the daughter should be able to successfully avoid pregnancy using the Ovulation Method.

The charts in Figures 5–4C and 5–4D show long cycles–from 37 to 51 days.

In long cycles there may be changes in hormonal activity that result in "patches of mucus," a succession of days of mucus secretion that interrupt the basic infertile pattern of either dry days or continuous mucous secretion. On such days, intercourse should not take place if pregnancy is being avoided because infertility cannot be assumed to be present.

CHARTING ANOVULATORY CYCLES

Figure 5–5 shows possibly anovulatory cycles in women from Australia, the United States, India, and Korea. It is possible for a woman to have one or more apparently anovulatory cycles a year (see Figure 5–5A–cycles 1 and 2; Figure 5–5B–all cycles; Figure 5–5C–cycles 1 and 2; Figure 5–5D–cycle 3; Figure 5–5E cycles 2, line 4; Figure 5–5F–cycles 4 and 6, lines 4 and 7).

Ordinarily, pregnancy ensues if intercourse occurs close to the time of ovulation.

Figure 5–3. The ovulatory phase can begin even during menstruation, as the white baby stamps early in the cycles indicate. *D.* Before learning the Ovulation Method, the woman had intercourse during menstruation, thinking that menstrual days were infertile ones. She became pregnant again and again. *F.* Brownish mucus that often appears before the menstrual flow.

Figure 5–4. Even women with long, irregular cycles can identify their fertile days by observing the mucous signs.

Figure 5-3

Short Cycles

A. Canada

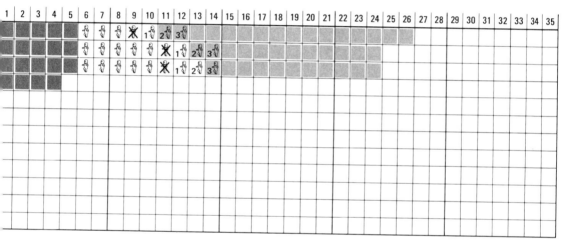

B. United States

C. Guatemala

NOTE: I = Intercourse

Figure 5-3 (continued)

Short Cycles (continued)

D. Mexico

1	2	3	4	5	6	7	8	9	10	11	12	13	14	15	16	17	18	19	20	21	22	23	24	25	26	27	28	29	30	31	32	33	34	35

E. Papua New Guinea

1	2	3	4	5	6	7	8	9	10	11	12	13	14	15	16	17	18	19	20	21	22	23	24	25	26	27	28	29	30	31	32	33	34	35

NOTE: I = Intercourse

F.

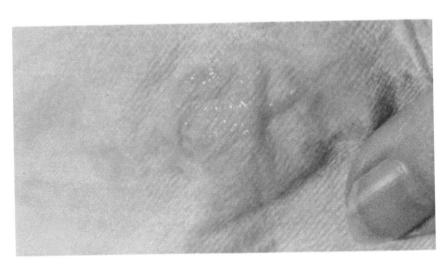

Irregular Cycles

Figure 5-4

A. Canada

B. Canada

C. Korea

D. Fiji

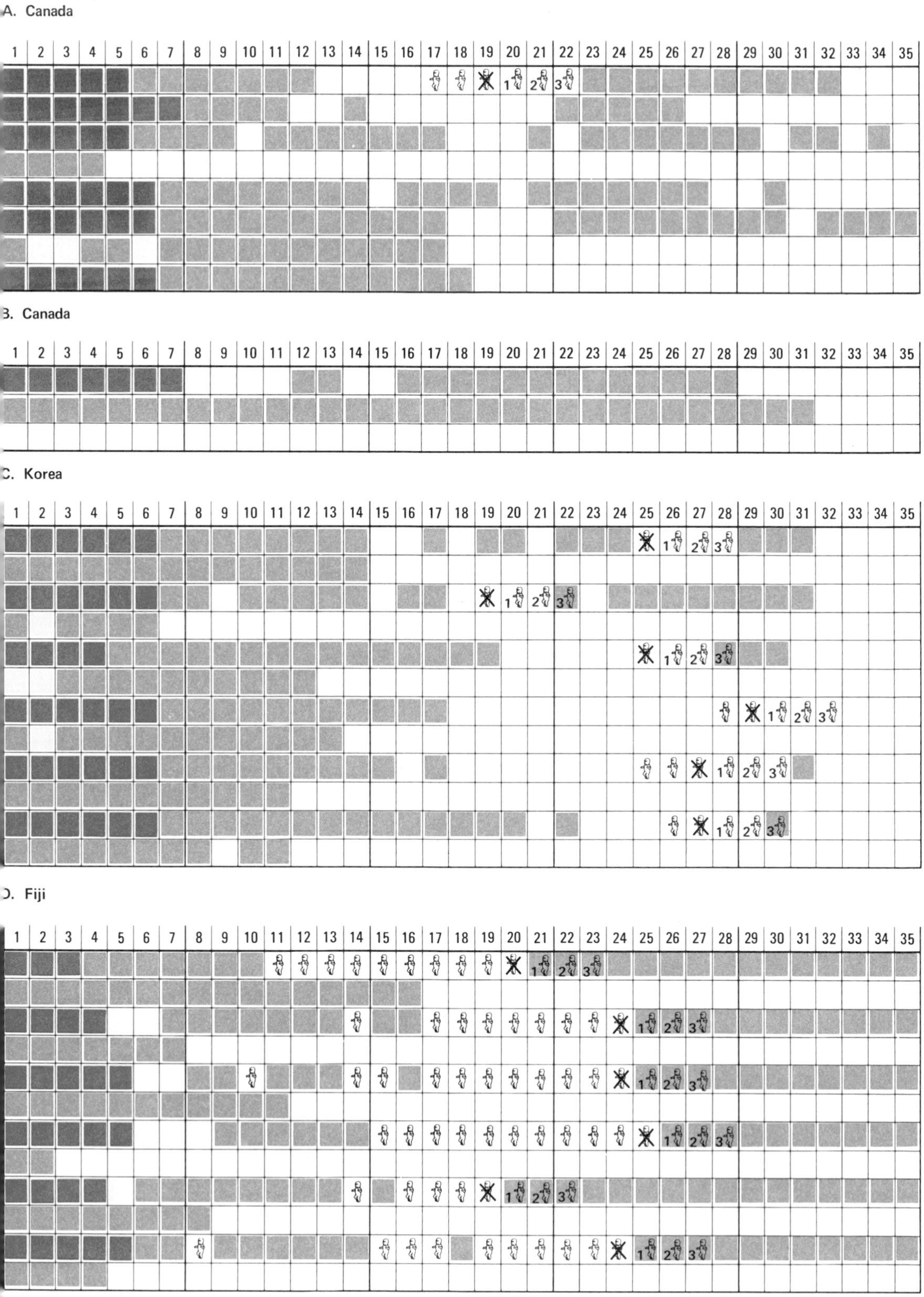

NOTE: I = Intercourse

If no mucus is present, however, intercourse close to the time of ovulation does not necessarily result in pregnancy. Two cases have been reported in which intercourse occurred close to the time of ovulation but did not result in pregnancy (page 90). The hormone levels indicated that ovulation had occurred, but the mucous signs did not. In both instances, the absence of mucus could explain why fertilization did not occur (page 92). The women involved were a premenopausal woman (page 92) and a young mother who was trying to become pregnant (Hilgers, 1977).

The chart shown in Figure 5–5A is that of a woman from Australia. She experienced bleeding on a regular basis in cycles 1 and 2. Mucus appeared one day each in cycles 1 and 2 (hence the white baby stamps), but the woman had no Peak day in either cycle. The short-lived mucous secretion could have been the result of estrogen levels at ovulation that were too low to reach a Peak. In the third cycle, the woman had a normal pattern of fertility and menstruation occurred two weeks later.

Figure 5–5B shows the chart of a young, unmarried nurse from the United States. Her mother had taught her to distinguish cloudy, sticky mucus from clear, elastic mucus. Throughout the year shown, the nurse had observed patches of sticky, cloudy mucus but never any clear, elastic mucus. Many nurses report irregular or apparently anovulatory cycles. Such cycles may be caused by the varying working and eating schedules many nurses have. In cycles of that type, the estrogen levels rise and fall as they do at ovulation during the normal cycles, but there is no luteal phase, or the luteal phase is very short and bleeding occurs as an estrogen-withdrawal phenomenon (breakthrough bleeding). Here the interval between the Peak day and menstruation was short. Cycles 2, 3, and 4 (particularly 3) in the chart shown in Figure 5–5B are excellent examples of that type of cycle.

Without knowledge of the hormone levels, cycles such as those just discussed cannot be considered absolutely anovulatory. Patches of clear, elastic mucus can occur sporadically in an apparently anovulatory cycle with constantly elevated estrogen levels that lead to breakthrough bleeding.

If there is any doubt about whether or not a cycle is truly anovulatory, the rules governing intercourse during the appearance of mucus must be observed (page 33).

Very young women often have irregular cycles. It is suspected that since they often diet, their menstrual irregularities are related to nutritional deficiencies. Pronounced irregularity and apparently anovulatory cycles are also often seen in records of women from communities in which nutrition is known to be poor. Those same records show, furthermore, that the women have relatively few days of the fertile mucous secretion. More studies of the possible relationship between nutrition and ovulation should be undertaken.

Irregular and apparently anovular cycles are common in young girls also because the reproductive organs and their interactions with the brain continue to mature during puberty. Thus it is important that young girls, especially, not be given the Pill, which could permanently alter the maturation process.

Figure 5–5. *A.* Possibly anovulatory cycles. Only if hormonal studies are done can it be determined whether or not ovulation occurred. *B.* The woman reported only infertile mucus. *C.* Breakthrough bleeding. *E.* The follicular phase lasted 66 days. *F.* Poor nutrition may have caused the reduction in the number of mucus days.

Figure 5–5   **Anovulatory (?) Cycles**

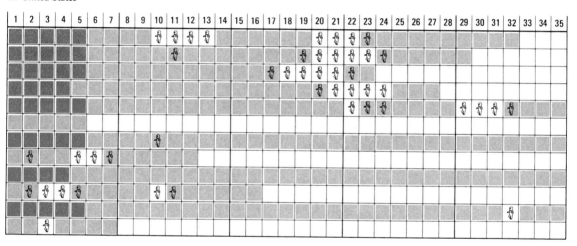

A. Australia

B. United States

C. India

NOTE: **I** = Intercourse

Figure 5-5 (continued)   **Anovulatory (?) Cycles (continued)**

D. Korea

E. United States

F. Korea

NOTE: **I** = Intercourse

The chart shown in Figure 5–4F is that of a 43-year-old Korean woman, a middle school graduate with three children. She had used the Rhythm Method in an attempt to regulate the number and spacing of her children, but she had had five unplanned pregnancies and five abortions. Note the small amount of mucus compared to the amount of mucus shown on charts of women from developed countries. Even though on her fourth cycle the woman did not have a second (later) appearance of mucus, she did not menstruate until 26 days after the first appearance of mucus. Probably there was not enough build-up of hormones to bring about a build-up of mucus, and the cycle was possibly anovulatory. The woman was tense while waiting for menstruation to occur, and it was hard to convince her that she was not pregnant. Fortunately, she took her teacher's advice to continue using alternative dry days for intercourse until other signs of pregnancy occurred. She was relieved when her menstrual period finally began.

Figure 5–5E shows the chart of a woman from the United States who had a very long cycle—ovulation occurred on the seventy-second day. In such a cycle, the Rhythm Method would have failed. If the woman had had intercourse close to the seventy-second day, the time of ovulation when many women report an increase in libido, she would probably have become pregnant.

A side benefit of the Ovulation Method is that in the case of pregnancy it can be used to pinpoint the date of conception. Thus even in the event of a long cycle, a pregnant woman and her doctor could estimate the delivery day (from the date of the last ovulation) with greater accuracy than they could calculating from the first day of the last menstrual period. Such precision reduces the chances that labor would be induced to deliver an only apparently overdue baby.

References

Billings, E.L., Billings, J.J., and Catarinich, M. Atlas of the Ovulation Method: The Mucus Patterns of Fertility and Infertility. Melbourne, Australia: Advocate Press, May 1977.

Hilgers, T.W. N.F.P. *Advocate,* July-August, 1977, Volume 2, Number 4.

6

Using the Ovulation Method to Achieve Pregnancy

The application of the Ovulation Method to help couples achieve pregnancy is the most recent important advance in the treatment of infertility (Billings 1977).

Couples who have been trying for 18 to 24 months to become pregnant are considered infertile. The investigation of the causes of their infertility is done systematically, and it includes history taking and physical examinations of both husband and wife, and the relevant laboratory tests, such as those to determine the patency of the fallopian tubes and to evaluate the quantity and quality of the sperm. Hormone and other studies are done to determine whether or not the woman is ovulating.

The Ovulation Method is easily applied to problems of infertility. Couples who wish to have children engage in intercourse when the mucous signs show that the woman is at her most fertile time.

The charts in this chapter are those of women from the United States, Australia, Korea, and India who were trying to have children. Some of the women were literate, some were not. As in all applications of the Ovulation Method, literacy is not necessary for success. Most of the charts are those of women who became pregnant after applying the Ovulation Method. The charts of the women who did not become pregnant show that the Ovulation Method can point out possible causes of the infertility.

Figure 6–1A shows the chart of an American woman who wanted to become pregnant and who did so twice in two years (the first pregnancy did not come to term). She was introduced to the Ovulation Method after five years of having taken the Pill. After four months of charting, she attempted to conceive. She did conceive (Figure

---

Figure 6–1. Intercourse close to the Peak day resulted in pregnancy.

Figure 6–2. *A.* In cycle 3, the woman had a normal build-up of mucus. Intercourse in that cycle resulted in pregnancy. *B.* The woman had intercourse when the mucus was alkaline–to increase her chances of conceiving a boy rather than a girl (see text). *C.* Hormone studies showed that ovulation occurred, but the woman did not become pregnant, probably because she did not have fertile mucus. *D.* Intercourse on the first day of fertile mucus resulted in pregnancy. *E.* Fertile mucus may be undetected during bleeding. Intercourse on a day of bleeding resulted in pregnancy. *F.* Hormone studies showed that ovulation occurred but the woman did not become pregnant, probably because she did not have fertile mucus.

For Achieving Pregnancy

1	2	3	4	5	6	7	8	9	10	11	12	13	14	15	16	17	18	19	20	21	22	23	24	25	26	27	28	29	30	31	32	33	34	35

Planned Pregnancy Followed by Miscarriage

1	2	3	4	5	6	7	8	9	10	11	12	13	14	15	16	17	18	19	20	21	22	23	24	25	26	27	28	29	30	31	32	33	34	35

1	2	3	4	5	6	7	8	9	10	11	12	13	14	15	16	17	18	19	20	21	22	23	24	25	26	27	28	29	30	31	32	33	34	35

NOTE: I = Intercourse

Figure 6-1 (continued)

For Achieving Pregnancy (continued)
United States

D.

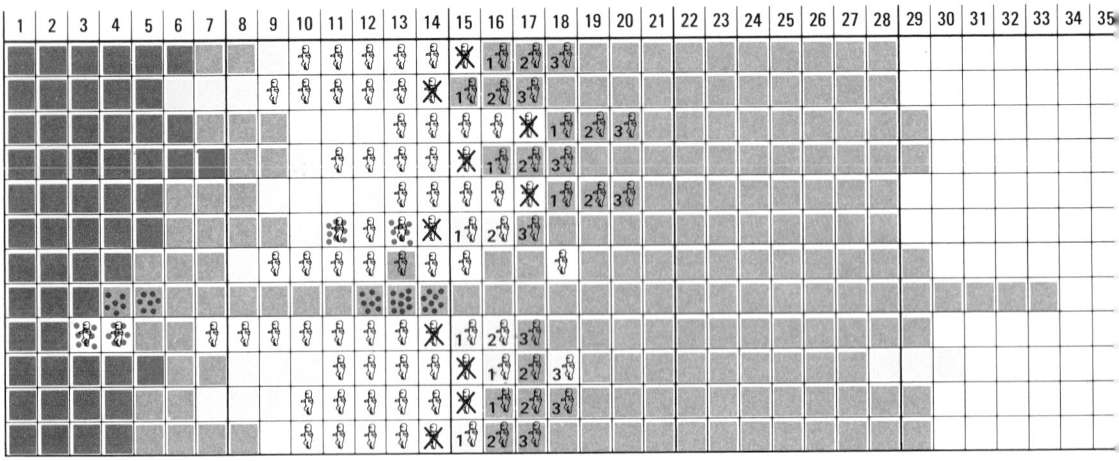

E.

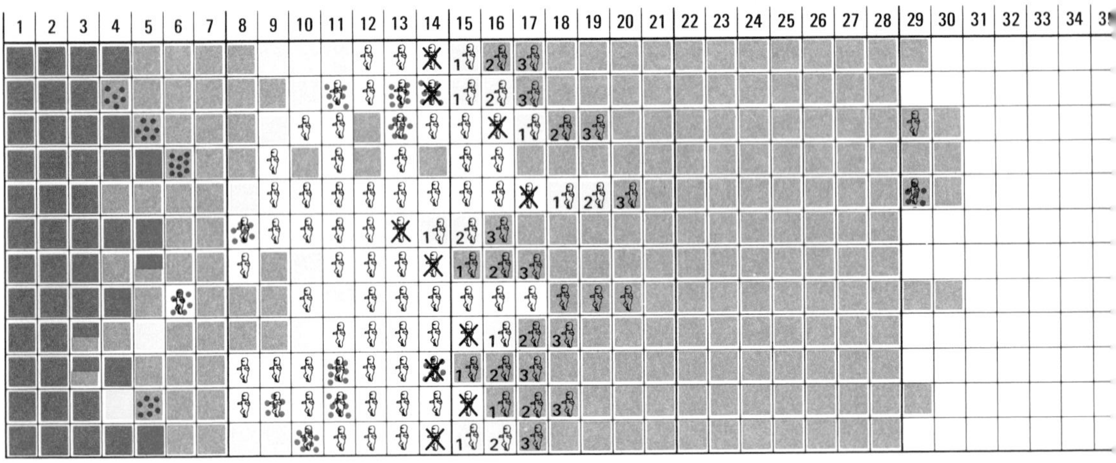

F.

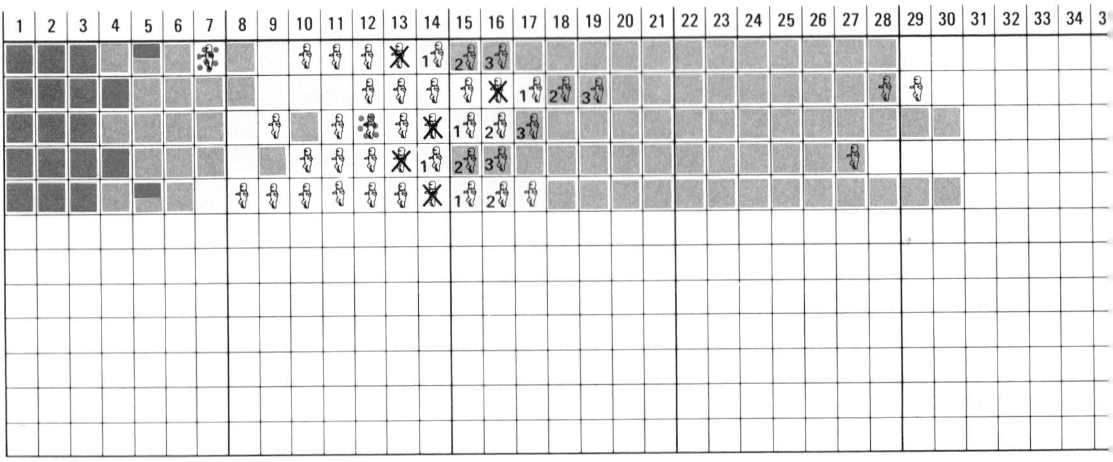

NOTE: **I** = Intercourse

Figure 6–2 **For Achieving Pregnancy**

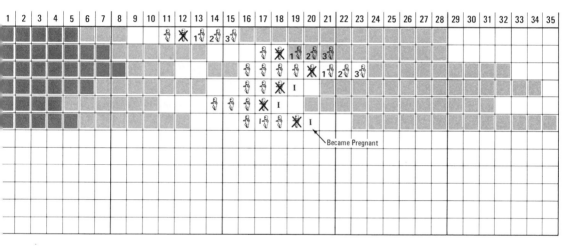

A. India

B. Korea

C. Australia

NOTE: **I** = Intercourse

D. Australia

1	2	3	4	5	6	7	8	9	10	11	12	13	14	15	16	17	18	19	20	21	22	23	24	25	26	27	28	29	30	31	32	33	34	35

E. Korea

1	2	3	4	5	6	7	8	9	10	11	12	13	14	15	16	17	18	19	20	21	22	23	24	25	26	27	28	29	30	31	32	33	34	35

Became pregnant

F. Australia

1	2	3	4	5	6	7	8	9	10	11	12	13	14	15	16	17	18	19	20	21	22	23	24	25	26	27	28	29	30	31	32	33	34	3*

NOTE: I = Intercourse

6–1A, Line 5), but she has a miscarriage. The miscarriage may have occurred because the pregnancy was her first one or because the uterus had not yet returned to normal after the long exposure to contraceptive steroids.

The woman again planned pregnancy and did indeed become pregnant—in the last cycle of the second year of charting (Fig. 6–1B, Line 12, Column 15). A healthy baby girl was born nine months later. The woman did not breast-feed, and she ovulated in the third cycle after childbirth (Figure 6–1C, Line 3). (For more detailed information about the rapid return of fertility after childbirth when the woman does not breastfeed, see pages 78 and 81.)

Note, in Figure 6–1B, the apparent absence of fertile mucus in cycles 2, 3 and 4 of the second year. The apparently anovulatory cycles coincided with the taking of antibiotics to counteract diarrhea. The same absense of fertile mucus was reported in her fourth year, Figure 6–1D, cycles 7 and 8 and her fifth year, Figure 6–1E, cycles 4 & 8 where the presence of influenza and/or the intake of medication may have been responsible for the possible anovulation. (For further information of the effects of illness and medication on ovulation, see Figure 7–2, p. 69).

Women who have been unable to conceive—and who on physical examination are shown to have no abnormalities—usually demonstrate a lack or sparcity of fertile mucus. The condition can sometimes be corrected by the establishment of good nutrition and the use of supplementary vitamins (page 49). If both these procedures are followed, fertile mucus may become evident—and in normal quantities.

Figure 6–2A shows the chart of a woman from India who wished to become pregnant. She also had a scanty mucous secretion in the first cycle after beginning the Ovulation Method. She had intercourse during the fertile-mucous days, (with no build-up of mucus before the fertile days). Even though she had intercourse during the fertile-mucous days, she did not become pregnant. In the second cycle, she had a normal mucus build-up, she had intercourse on the Peak day, and she became pregnant.

Figure 6–2B shows how a woman (from Korea) who had two daughters used the Ovulation Method to conceive a son rather than a daughter.

If a sperm containing an X chromosome unites with the ovum, a female will be conceived, whereas if a sperm containing a Y chromosome unites with the ovum, a male will be conceived. Since (it is theorized) X-containing sperm are stronger and survive longer than do Y-containing sperm, couples wishing to have a girl should have intercourse when the mucus is slightly acid, at the time of transition from infertile to fertile mucus. The acid environment would destroy more Y-containing sperm than X-containing sperm and thus would enhance the possibility that the woman would conceive a female. If the couple wishes to have a boy, they should have intercourse when the mucus is alkaline, that is, at the Peak, the last day of clear-stretchy mucus. Since alkaline mucus promotes the survival of all sperm and since the Y-containing sperm apparently move faster, it is likely that the Y-containing sperm would reach the ovum first.

As shown in the chart in Figure 6–2B, intercourse took place just before and just after Peak in the sixth cycle. The woman conceived and had a son. In cycles 4 and 5, probably too eager to succeed, the woman had intercourse after the Peak day, and she did not conceive. As mentioned elsewhere, if sperm are present for a number of hours before ovulation, the chances that the woman will get pregnant are enhanced.

Figure 6–2C shows the chart of a 30-year-old woman from Australia who for several years had been trying to get pregnant. She had even tried artificial insemination. Hormone studies covering two cycles showed that ovulation had occurred. However, the woman stated that the mucus secretions were always of the infertile type. She also had cervical erosion, retroversion on the uterus, and cysts on both ovaries. The cysts were removed. About a year later, the woman reported fertile mucus in two cycles, giving hope that she might yet become pregnant.

Figure 6–2D shows the chart of an Australian woman. Scanty, fertile mucus was observed only for a couple of hours in the morning, as shown in cycle 2, column 17. Intercourse during the fertile hours resulted in pregnancy. Note that only infertile mucus appeared in cycle 1 and that repeated attempts to become pregnant had failed. It should be remembered that sperm survive in the reproductive tract for a number of hours as they move toward the ovum. Since fertile mucus assists in the transport and survival of sperm, to be maximally effective in achieving pregnancy, intercourse should take place just before ovulation. If this couple had waited until the evening to have intercourse, chances are that conception would not have occurred as the elevation of progesterone that afternoon would have changed the mucus characteristic to the infertile type, obstructing the penetration of the sperm.

Figure 6–2E shows the chart of a 30-year-old Korean woman. (She was illiterate.) When she was introduced to the Ovulation Method, she claimed that she had never observed fertile mucus. After using the Ovulation Method successfully for six months, she began to question whether she was ovulating. In the sixth cycle, column 15, she had intercourse on the second day of some spotting and became pregnant.

The fact that the woman's mucous secretion was scanty may reflect her diet. She never ate meat or eggs; she ate fish rarely, perhaps once every two months. Her main diet was rice with pickled vegetables, which she ate three times a day. Poor nutrition and poor living conditions seem to have adverse effects on mucous secretions (pages 54, 55 and 56).

Figure 6–2F shows the chart of a woman from Australia who for eight years had been trying to get pregnant. Hormone studies proved that ovulation had occurred in cycles 4, 5, and 6. The woman stated that she had not had any clear, elastic mucus for a number of years. She also had had cysts removed from both ovaries. Perhaps the absence of fertile mucus or the cysts (or both) caused the infertility.

REFERENCES

Billings, E.L., Billings, J.J. and Catarinich, M. *Atlas of the Ovulation Method: The Mucus Patterns of Fertility and Infertility,* Melbourne, Australia: Advocate Press, May, 1977.

7

Emotional and Physical States that Affect the Mucous Secretion (Tension, Illness, Medication, Childbirth, Breast-feeding, the Menopause)

Chapter 7 discusses alterations of the mucous secretion that are associated with various emotional and physical states—alterations associated with physical and mental stress, illness, medication, childbirth (in both the woman who is breast-feeding and the one who is not), and during the menopausal years.

Since ovulation involves the synchronous functioning of several organs—the brain, pituitary, and ovaries—it is not surprising that the ovulatory process can be altered temporarily by the use of drugs or by illness itself. Psychological disturbances and dramatic changes in lifestyle may also disrupt the synchrony of events that lead to ovulation. Furthermore, permanent suspension of ovulation has been reported as a result of the prolonged use of the Pill (see pages 95–96).

EFFECT OF TENSION ON OVULATION

In Figure 7–1 ovulation records from women in the United States and Australia— ovulation was shown to have been delayed from one to five months during periods of tension and psychological unrest.

Figure 7–1A shows the chart of a young woman whose ovulatory patterns were normal for the first four cycles. In the fifth cycle, the mucus build-up and ovulation were interrupted by a traumatic event. Her fiance returned from Vietnam and differences of opinion emerged at that time resulting in a broken engagement. Judging by the absence of fertile mucus, it is presumed that this traumatic condition continued to influence her irregularity indefinitely in the following cycles.

Figure 7–1B shows the chart of a young American teen-ager. She had been charting accurately for two years and had even been teaching the Ovulation Method to other teen-agers. When she went away to college (during the cycle 3), her normal ovulatory pattern was disrupted so that only cloudy, sticky mucus, not clear, elastic mucus, was seen. As the young woman became adjusted to her new life, the cycles returned to normal. Irregularity of cycles is quite common in young women when they leave home for college or to lead another type of life. The irregularity is usually temporary, and the cycles return to normal within a few months.

Figure 7–1C shows the chart of an American woman, the mother of one child. She began charting shortly after discontinuing the Pill, which she had taken for six months. Note the extended period of mucous secretion. In spite of the secretion she was able to distinguish cloudy, sticky mucus from clear, elastic mucus and thus to determine when ovulation occurred. Such an extended secretion frequently occurs after discontinuation of the Pill (pages 95 to 98). The woman's succeeding cycles were fairly regular, as indicated by recognition of the Peak days.

During the fifth cycle, the couple had marital problems. This situation was magnified when the husband lost his job. Immediately thereafter, the wife had mostly cloudy, sticky mucus for 78 days after her menstrual period. Following this ordeal when the husband found a steady job and their relations normalized, the mucus almost immediately became clear and elastic (line 7) and was accompanied by spotting.

As happened in the case just described, when ovulation has been postponed, a slight bleeding may accompany the appearance of clear, elastic mucus, after a long period of infertility. For that reason, women should be warned that when mucus has been observed—even though bleeding occurred—ovulation has probably taken place and a true menstrual period will probably follow in about two weeks. That was the case with the woman whose chart is shown in Figure 7–1C. Menstruation occurred about 14 days after the appearance of clear, elastic mucus. The stability in her personal life is reflected in the regular cycles that followed in the year and a half shown on the chart.

The chart in Figure 7–1D belongs to a 45-year-old premenopausal Australian woman, and shows how stress from various causes affected her cycles. Hormone studies confirmed that ovulation did not occur. She is a mother of five children and had been on the Ovulation Method for six years. She had always had regular cycles. At this time she was participating in a project studying the effectiveness of the Ovulation Method in premenopausal women, and was asked to keep a record of her temperature. She experienced continuous mucus which she described as a "white smear." This was her basic infertile pattern which she was quite familiar with.

Figure 7–1. *A.* Broken engagement (cycle 5). *B.* Abrupt change of lifestyle when the girl went away to college. *C.* Marital and job problems (cycle 5). *D.* Stress in a premenopausal woman. Hormone studies showed that ovulation did not occur, despite the rise in basal body temperature.

Figure 7–2. *A.* Tension and/or medication may have delayed normal mucus build-up *B.* Ovulation was delayed by illness. The woman disregarded the rules and became pregnant. *C.* Measles may have delayed the normal mucus build-up in cycle 2. *D.* A cervical ulcer, which was cauterized, may have caused the reduction in the number of days of fertile mucus (cycles 3, 4, and 5). *E.* A vaginal infection— or the medication taken to cure it—may have caused the absence of fertile mucus. *F.* An ovarian cyst may have caused the disturbances in the mucus pattern.

Figure 7-1   Tension can delay Ovulation

A. United States broken engagement cycles

| 1 | 2 | 3 | 4 | 5 | 6 | 7 | 8 | 9 | 10 | 11 | 12 | 13 | 14 | 15 | 16 | 17 | 18 | 19 | 20 | 21 | 22 | 23 | 24 | 25 | 26 | 27 | 28 | 29 | 30 | 31 | 32 | 33 | 34 | 35 |

B. United States adjustment to college

| 1 | 2 | 3 | 4 | 5 | 6 | 7 | 8 | 9 | 10 | 11 | 12 | 13 | 14 | 15 | 16 | 17 | 18 | 19 | 20 | 21 | 22 | 23 | 24 | 25 | 26 | 27 | 28 | 29 | 30 | 31 | 32 | 33 | 34 | 35 |

NOTE: I = Intercourse

Figure 7-1 (continued)   Tension can delay Ovulation (continued)

C. United States marital discord. Job problem cycles

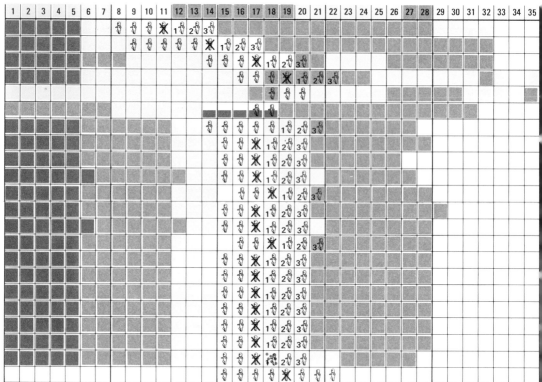

NOTE: I = Intercourse

D. Stress in pre-menopausal years

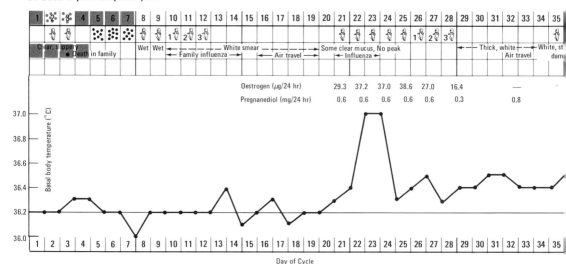

Day of Cycle

Figure 7-2

Medication and (or) Illness can Delay Ovulation

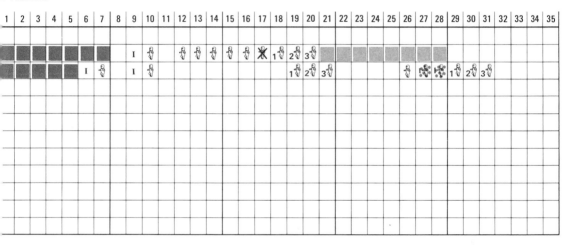

A. Australia

B. Australia

C. United States

NOTE: I = Intercourse

D. Mexico

E. Korea

F. Australia

NOTE: **I** = Intercourse

In this particular cycle several traumatic events occurred. A relative died on day 3 of her cycle. Her family developed influenza, and in the third week she had to travel. In the second week the mucus changed from her basic infertile pattern on days 9 and 10. On day 21 some fertile mucus was encountered but at the same time she also came down with the flu. Five days later she reverted to her usual basic infertile pattern without a defined peak. The cycle finished without ovulation, as was subsequently confirmed by hormonal assays.

The temperature rise occurred while she had the flu, and remained elevated even after her recovery and despite the fact that ovulation did not take place on that particular cycle.

THE EFFECT OF MEDICATION AND ILLNESS ON OVULATION

The evidence seems to show that illness or medication (or both) can delay ovulation for a few days or for several cycles. Women learning the Ovulation Method should be made aware of that possibility, even though medication may not always delay ovulation, since the reaction to medication is individual. The examples shown in Figure 7-2 indicate (1) the effect medication had on some women; and (2) that those women were still able to recognize their fertile period.

Figure 7-2A shows the chart of an Australian woman who had successfully used the Ovulation Method to avoid pregnancy. In her third cycle, ovulation was postponed, probably because of tension or medication (or both). The ovulatory phase had begun normally enough. Then the woman's child had an attack of asthma for the first time, a relative died, and the woman took medicine for hay fever. In accordance with the rules, the woman avoided intercourse for three days after the first appearance of the mucus. Her teacher warned her that since she had not seen clear, elastic mucus she must watch for a possible return of mucus. Five days later, mucus returned, with two days of clear, elastic mucus. Ovulation probably took place at that time since the next menstrual period occurred two weeks later.

The baby stamps in the pre-ovulatory phase of cycles 1, 3, 4 and 5 do not necessarily mean that clear, elastic mucus was present. Seminal fluid deposited in the vaginal canal during intercourse is often discharged the next morning, and it resembles clear elastic mucus. Although with experience most women can distinguish seminal fluid from mucous secretion, those who cannot should avoid intercourse the day after intercourse (page 33, footnote).

In the chart shown in Figure 7-2B from Australia, ovulation was shown also to have been delayed following an illness (cycle 2), with clear, elastic mucus appearing late in the same cycle. Even though this woman had been warned to avoid intercourse if fertile mucus would appear late in the cycle following illness or medication, she disregarded the rules, had intercourse when fertile mucus was present accompanied by slight bleeding and became pregnant.

Women who become ill or who take medicine at the beginning of the ovulatory phase of the cycle must follow the rules for intercourse during times of mucous secretion or bleeding. Ovulation that has been delayed may occur late in the cycle. Each cycle must be treated separately and without reference to the previous one.

Figure 7–2C shows the chart of an 18-year-old American woman. The shortness of her luteal phases made her teacher wonder if she was ovulating at all. However, the normal pattern of her mucous secretions shows that ovulation may have occurred. The woman's second cycle was an unusually long one, and on the forty-second day of that cycle she reported the outbreak of measles. Note that fertile mucus did not occur until the illness had ended. The incubation period for measles is about three weeks. Thus, it can be assumed that in this one case the mucous secretion and/or ovulation were suspended from the beginning of the incubation period until the end of the illness.

The chart of a Mexican woman (illiterate) shown in Figure 7–2D illustrates how illness can affect ovulation. After having had two normal cyles, the woman had an ulcer that was cauterized. Infertility coincided with the period of illness, hospitalization and medication (cycles 3, 4 and 5). Successive cycles were normal.

The chart of the Korean woman (Figure 7–2E) shows a continuous discharge of cloudy, sticky mucus that was associated with a vaginal infection, or with the medicine used to cure the infection, or with both. In such cases, the woman must determine what is her basic infertile pattern (pages 36–37). If she observes any change in the quantity or quality of the mucous secretion, she must avoid intercourse from the day of the change until the fourth day after her return to the basic infertile pattern. Furthermore, in five out of nine cycles, ovulation possibly did not occur. Poor nutrition may have contributed to the irregularity. The woman's diet consisted of poor quality rice and vegetables. She rarely ate fish, and she never ate meat.

A most important point to be mentioned about the advantages of the Ovulation Method is the ability of the woman to detect some gynaecological disturbances. Abnormalities that are recorded in the charting indicate quite obviously that something is wrong. This can be vaginal or uterine infections, tumors, endometriosis, cervical erosions or uterine cancer, to name a few. Abnormalities in her normal pattern will alert her to seek medical help. Figure 7–2F belongs to a young woman who had been married about two years and had been following the Ovulation Method to avoid pregnancy, until they decided to start a family. She developed a strange pattern in her normal mucous pattern which was later found to have been caused by a cyst in the ovary. In the second cycle they tried to achieve pregnancy and when menstruation did not follow, the wife went to her physician for a pregnancy test. The test was negative. Several weeks afterwards, as you can clearly see from her chart, a disturbed mucous pattern and irregular bleeding was encountered. She went to her gynaecologist who found an ovarian cyst and had it removed. After the cyst was removed, bleeding followed as well as patches of mucus without a definite peak. In the last cycle, the couple used the day of Peak for intercourse, but did not achieve pregnancy.

Figure 7–3. *A.* Medication or illness sometimes does not affect the mucus pattern, as this three-year record shows. *C.* Hypertension developed (cycle 9). *D.* Fibroid tumors of the uterus.

Figure 7–4. Even women with discharges can tell when they are fertile, *A, C, D.* The women could recognize the change to fertile mucus. *B.* The women could recognize the Peak day. *E.* The infertile mucous discharge often observed in the postovulatory phase of the cycle and the chronic noninfectious discharge are similar in appearance.

Figure 7-3

Medication and (or) Illness may not Delay Ovulation
United States—Three Year Records

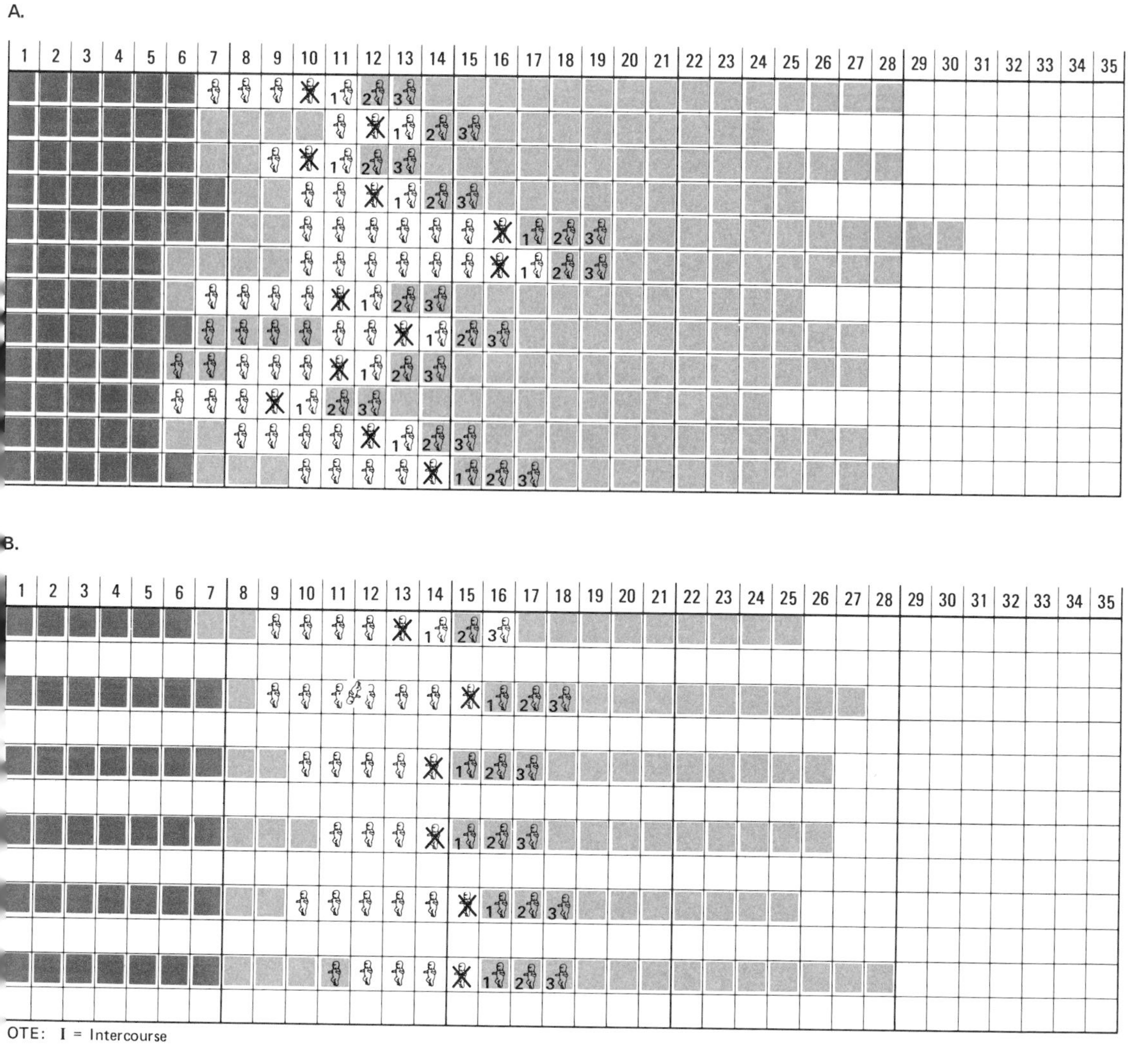

OTE: **I** = Intercourse

C.

1	2	3	4	5	6	7	8	9	10	11	12	13	14	15	16	17	18	19	20	21	22	23	24	25	26	27	28	29	30	31	32	33	34	35

D. Uterine Fibroids did not Affect her Regularity

1	2	3	4	5	6	7	8	9	10	11	12	13	14	15	16	17	18	19	20	21	22	23	24	25	26	27	28	29	30	31	32	33	34	35

NOTE: I = Intercourse

Figure 7-4

Recognizing Fertile Mucus Despite a Non-Infectious or an Infectious Discharge

A. United States

1	2	3	4	5	6	7	8	9	10	11	12	13	14	15	16	17	18	19	20	21	22	23	24	25	26	27	28	29	30	31	32	33	34	35

B. Mexico

1	2	3	4	5	6	7	8	9	10	11	12	13	14	15	16	17	18	19	20	21	22	23	24	25	26	27	28	29	30	31	32	33	34	35

NOTE: **I** = Intercourse

Figure 7-4
(continued)

Recognizing Fertile Mucus Despite a Non-Infectious or an Infectious Discharge (continued)

C. United States

1	2	3	4	5	6	7	8	9	10	11	12	13	14	15	16	17	18	19	20	21	22	23	24	25	26	27	28	29	30	31	32	33	34	35

D. Dominican Republic

1	2	3	4	5	6	7	8	9	10	11	12	13	14	15	16	17	18	19	20	21	22	23	24	25	26	27	28	29	30	31	32	33	34	35

NOTE: I = Intercourse

E.

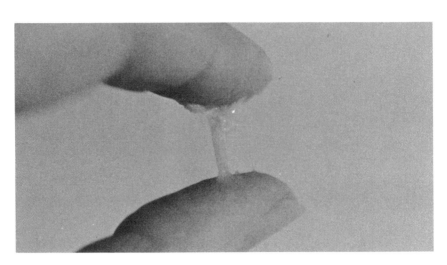

A more dramatic event of this nature was recently reported to the author. A mother of five in her forties who previously had been on the pill for nine years and was introduced to the Ovulation Method six years ago found that something was wrong by the appearance of unusual mucus and bleeding. A previous pap smear did not reveal any abnormality, in fact, she had had a negative pap smear two months before. The Ob/Gyn doctor took a tissue biopsy just to humor her apprehension and was surprised to find a precancerous condition in the uterus. She subsequently had a vaginal hysterectomy.

Figure 7–3 shows that medication and/or illness do not always affect ovulation. The chart is that of an American woman. In the second year of charting, she developed hypertension, but that condition did not affect the regularity of her cycles. Fibroid tumors of the uterus were detected in the middle of her third year of charting. They also did not affect her cycles. Eventually the woman had a partial hysterectomy. Since the operation she has not had a clear, elastic mucous secretion (Figure 7–3, page 73) only a slight, cloudy, sticky one.

CHRONIC, NONINFECTIOUS DISCHARGES; ACUTE, INFECTIOUS DISCHARGES

Figure 7–4 shows the charts of four women who had either chronic, noninfectious discharges or acute infectious discharges (Figure 7–4E). A woman who has either type of discharge is nevertheless able to distinguish clear, elastic mucus from the discharge, an ability doctors often question.

Figure 7–4A shows the chart of an American woman who had a chronic, noninfectious discharge that was similar in amount every day until the ovulatory phase began, when the amount of mucus increased and its consistency changed. Those changes gave ample warning that ovulation was beginning and that intercourse should be avoided from the day of the changes until the fourth day after the return to the basic infertile pattern (see page 36). Reports from women from different cultures with similar discharges state that they too can tell when the ovulatory phase begins because the mucus increases in quantity. The normal mucous secretion and the discharge are different in color and elasticity—the chronic or infectious discharge does not stretch, whereas the mucous secretion does. Therefore, the presence of a discharge creates no problem in pinpointing the fertile phase of her cycle. The green stamps encoded with the letter M indicated that even though there was a discharge, it was an infertile one and the day was a safe (infertile) day.

Figure 7–4B shows the chart of a Mexican woman (illiterate) who had an infectious discharge at the time she started charting. But she was able to distinguish clear, elastic mucus from the infectious discharge even in the first cycle. When the woman was given medication, the infectious discharge diminished. Again the woman was able to pinpoint the time of ovulation. Her cycles returned to normal, and the discharge was considerably reduced after the infection disappeared (cycle 4).

The chart in Figure 7–4C, which is similar to the one in Figure 7–4A shows that the woman was able to distinguish her fertile phase without any doubt from her chronic noninfectious discharge.

The chart shown in Figure 7–4D is that of a woman from the Dominican Republic who began charting at the age of 40. She had seven children (and had had one miscarriage). Although she had a chronic, noninfectious discharge in every cycle she could detect the change to clear, elastic mucus and then back to her basic infertile pattern.

Figure 7–4E shows the mucus of a chronic noninfectious discharge. It is similar in appearance to the infertile mucus often observed in the postovulatory phase of the cycle.

INTERCOURSE DURING THE EARLY SAFE DAYS

After using the Ovulation Method for a time, some couples decide that they want to have another child. Such couples are able to experiment in the preovulatory phase of their cycle to test how close to peak they can have intercourse without becoming pregnant. The information will be useful later on in possibly reducing the number of abstinence days.

As shown in the chart in Figure 7–5A, intercourse that took place on the second day of the mucous secretion of cycles 5 and 6 did not result in pregnancy. In the following cycle, not shown, intercourse occurred in the later days of the mucous secretion, when the mucus had changed from cloudy, sticky mucus to clear, elastic mucus, resulting in pregnancy.

Figure 7–5B shows the chart of an American woman. The couple concerned were eager to have a child, and they also wanted to test the Ovulation Method in the first few cycles so that in the future they would know approximately how many days of cloudy, sticky mucus they could later use for intercourse without the risk of pregnancy. In the first cycle, intercourse took place up to the third and fourth days of the mucous secretion, just two days short of the Peak day. In the third cycle, intercourse took place on the first day of the mucous secretion, two days before the Peak day. In the fourth cycle, there was a minimum build-up of mucus, with no Peak day (the cycle was perhaps anovulatory). In the last cycle, intercourse took place on the Peak day, and the woman became pregnant.

The chart in Figure 7–5C shows that intercourse on the second day of the mucous secretion did not result in pregnancy.[1] However, this is not a recommended policy for those couples wishing to postpone pregnancy, temporarily or permanently.

OVULATION AFTER CHILDBIRTH

Ovulation in the Woman Who is not Breast-feeding Her Baby

Women who do not breast-feed their babies return to normal ovulatory patterns within a cycle or two after childbirth.

Figure 7–5. *A.* Intercourse on the second day of the mucous secretion did not result in pregnancy. *B.* Intercourse took place on Peak day, and pregnancy resulted. *C.* Intercourse on the second day of the mucous secretion did not result in pregnancy.

---

[1] These examples are illustrative of the fact that for successful induction of pregnancy, intercourse should occur close to the time of presumed ovulation.

Testing the Fertility of Cloudy, Sticky, Mucus

United States

2	3	4	5	6	7	8	9	10	11	12	13	14	15	16	17	18	19	20	21	22	23	24	25	26	27	28	29	30	31	32	33	34	35

United States

2	3	4	5	6	7	8	9	10	11	12	13	14	15	16	17	18	19	20	21	22	23	24	25	26	27	28	29	30	31	32	33	34	35

Canada

2	3	4	5	6	7	8	9	10	11	12	13	14	15	16	17	18	19	20	21	22	23	24	25	26	27	28	29	30	31	32	33	34	35

TE: I = Intercourse

Ovulation usually occurs before the first menstrual flow after childbirth. If the woman has been accurately instructed, she can pinpoint not only the time of ovulation, but also the approximate date of her menstrual flow (two weeks later). Sometimes the cycle after the first fertile cycle is irregular or anovular.

The three charts shown in Figure 7–6 are those of women from Canada, U.S.A. and Mexico who began charting after the lochia ended, (the lochia is the vaginal discharge that normally occurs in the weeks after childbirth). The mucous secretion appeared soon afterward. The Peak day was recognized and the menstrual period began two weeks later.

The Chart shown in Figure 7–6B shows that an apparently anovulatory cycle occurred in the cycle after the first fertile postpartum cycle.

Ovulation in the Woman Who is Breast-feeding Her Baby

The Ovulation Method is particularly suitable for the woman who is breast-feeding because it enables her to recognize infertility even though she is not ovulating. Thus there is usually no need to wean the baby so that ovulation will be restored.

Many months can pass until the first menstruation occurs; the exact dates of the return of ovulation and menstruation cannot be predicted. The dates of return depend on the general health of the woman, and on whether or not she is "totally breast-feeding" her baby (the term totally means that the child is receiving no other nourishment than the mother's milk). It is unusual for fertility to return when a baby is being totally breast-fed for the first three months.

After the lochia has stopped, there is usually a period of dryness. At that point, the woman begins to chart.

The chart shown in Figure 7–7A is that of a 23-year old American woman who was breast-feeding her second child. The baby was totally breast-fed for six months, and was then introduced to solid foods (line 4). The first mucous secretions appeared at the same time. When a baby is introduced to solids, his appetite decreases, and as a result the stimulation of the mother's pituitary gland that his suckling produces is diminished. The woman's first apparent fertile cycle occurred when the baby was 17 months old (line 15). The baby was still breast-feeding at 21 months, even though the woman's menstrual periods had returned. The Peak day was indicated by an x on the white baby stamp.

Abstinence if dryness exists continuously during the nursing period is not required. The rules for intercourse during the weaning period are the same for nursing mothers who have not yet ovulated as for any other woman experiencing the pre-ovulatory phase. If one day of cloudy sticky mucus is observed, intercourse should be avoided that day plus three more days restricting intercourse to the evenings during the weaning period (dry day, safe night). After ovulation has been observed as in the case of 7–7A, the post-ovulatory rules will apply, i.e. if one day of sticky, tacky mu-

---

Figure 7-6. The women observed the first appearance of fertile mucus and thus were able to predict when menstruation would return.

Figure 7-6

Return to Fertility After Childbirth in Women not Breastfeeding

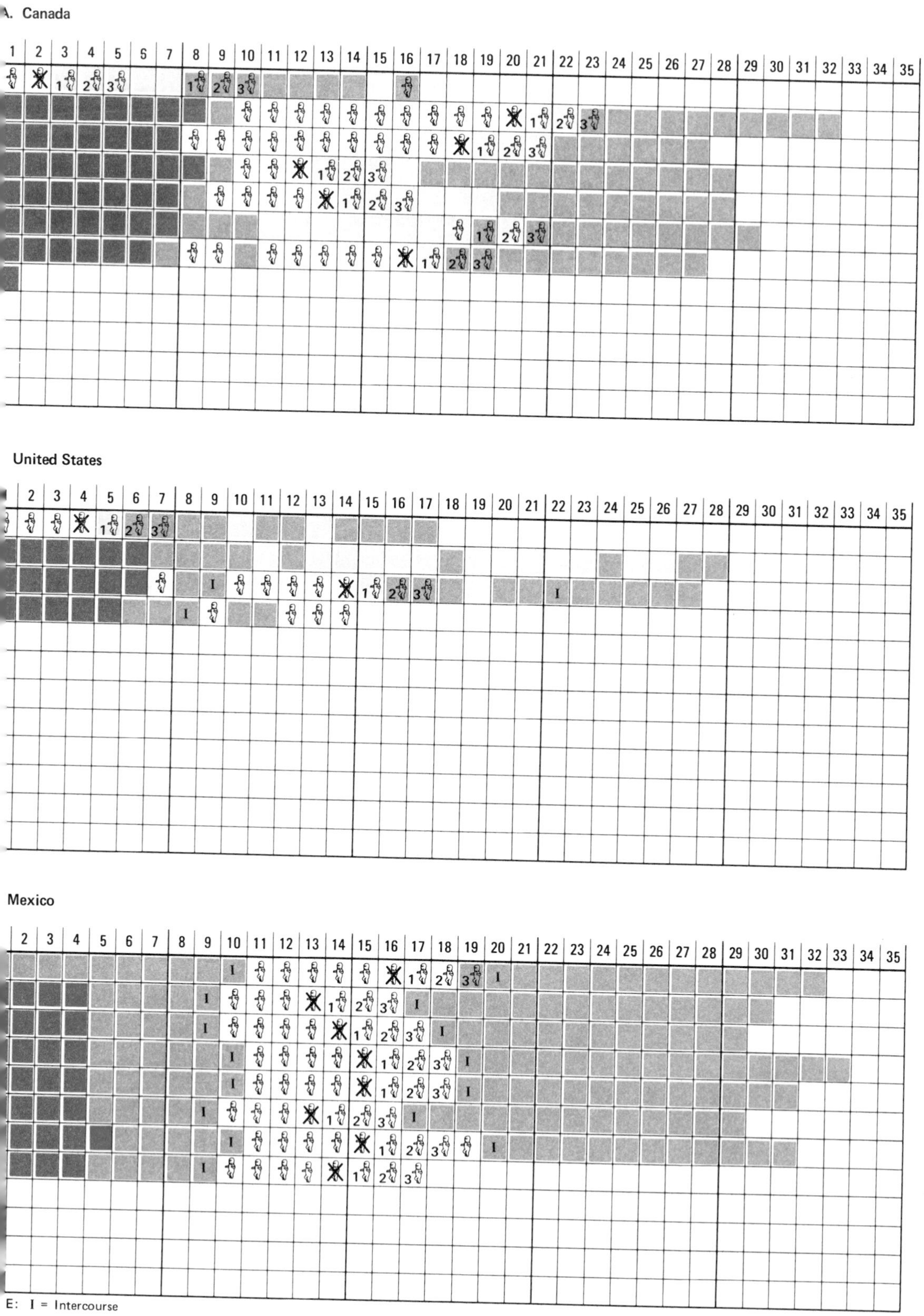

A. Canada

United States

Mexico

E: I = Intercourse

cus is observed intercourse must be avoided on that day. If the next day is dry, intercourse can be resumed. If two days of sticky, tacky mucus are observed the same rule applies. However, if three days of this type mucus is observed it is advisable to abstain three extra dry days before resuming intercourse. Occasionally nursing mothers have only one day of clear, elastic mucus and then dryness. Such women must avoid intercourse that day plus three more days of dryness. Sometimes nursing mothers also experience a continued sensation of wetness. Again, caution is advised by avoiding those days plus three extra days.

Figure 7–7B shows the chart of an American woman who was nursing her fourth child. She began charting after the baby was born. The red stamps indicate the lochia. The two baby stamps in the first line indicate the appearance of sticky mucus, which coincided with the time that the baby had an ear infection and was breast-feeding less. As explained, the stimulation provided by a baby sucking is believed to inhibit ovulation. Note how quickly the mucus appeared when breast-feeding decreased. A similar situation was encountered when the baby was introduced to solid foods (line 7). Line 8 shows a normal ovulatory pattern as breast-feedings continue to decrease. The luteal phase was longer than normal, a common occurrence in nursing mothers. In the last cycle the woman had no fertile mucus, probably because she had a viral infection for which she was taking medicine.

The chart shown in Figure 7–7C is that of a 26-year-old woman from Papua New Guinea who had three children. Her diet was good, and she was reasonably healthy. Complete dryness was present through the breast-feeding period and that as weaning began, patches of mucus appeared and a normal pattern was re-established quite rapidly.

The chart shown in Figure 7–7D is that of an illiterate Mexican woman, the mother of nine children. She started charting when she began to wean her baby. Patches of infertile mucus appeared, then she was able to pinpoint her first fertile cycle (line 2). Her menstrual periods were quite normal after that.

The chart shown in Figure 7–7E is that of a 22-year-old illiterate Nigerian woman who had a three-month-old baby. The woman's diet was good. The long periods of dryness and the occasional small patches of infertile mucus in the first two months of nursing are typical for nursing mothers.

Figure 7–7. *A.* While totally breast-feeding her baby, the woman had no mucous secretion. The mucous secretion started when she began to wean her baby. *B.* A mucous patch occurred in the first month when the baby was ill and feeding poorly and when the baby was introduced to solids (line 7). Fertile mucus first appeared in the seventh month (line 9). A viral illness and/or medication delayed the appearance of fertile mucus in the last cycle. *C.* While totally breast-feeding the baby, the woman had no mucous secretion. The secretion started two weeks before the first menstrual period. *D.* The patches of mucous first appeared when the woman began to wean her baby. Her menstrual periods soon re-established themselves. *E.* Long periods of dryness were broken by occasional patches of mucus. *F.* Hormone studies showed that clear, elastic mucus coincided with an increase in the woman's blood levels of estrogens *(heavy lines)*. *G.* Patches of mucus appeared when the woman was weaning her baby. *H.* Hormone studies confirmed that ovulation coincided with the appearance of fertile mucus when the woman was weaning her baby. *I.* Various changes that occurred in a woman that nursed her child for two years. *J.* Fertility returned 6 weeks after childbirth even though the woman was totally breast-feeding. *K.* The milky discharge that is often present in nursing mothers

Return to Fertility in Nursing Mothers

a. United States

United States

Solids introduced

NOTE: **I** = Intercourse

C. Papua New Guinea

D. Mexico

E. Nigeria

NOTE: **I** = Intercourse

Return to Fertility in Nursing Mothers (continued)

Australia

| 2 | 3 | 4 | 5 | 6 | 7 | 8 | 9 | 10 | 11 | 12 | 13 | 14 | 15 | 16 | 17 | 18 | 19 | 20 | 21 | 22 | 23 | 24 | 25 | 26 | 27 | 28 | 29 | 30 | 31 | 32 | 33 | 34 | 35 |

← Vacationing →

Vacationing

India

| 2 | 3 | 4 | 5 | 6 | 7 | 8 | 9 | 10 | 11 | 12 | 13 | 14 | 15 | 16 | 17 | 18 | 19 | 20 | 21 | 22 | 23 | 24 | 25 | 26 | 27 | 28 | 29 | 30 | 31 | 32 | 33 | 34 | 35 |

Australia

| 1 | 2 | 3 | 4 | 5 | 6 | 7 | 8 | 9 | 10 | 11 | 12 | 13 | 14 | 15 | 16 | 17 | 18 | 19 | 20 | 21 | 22 | 23 | 24 | 25 | 26 | 27 | 28 | 29 | 30 | 31 | 32 | 33 | 34 | 35 |

Baby, 3½ months; fully breast-feeding, 5 feeds daily

1 teaspoon cereal

← Slight mucus →

← Tacky, sticky, mucus →

Children sick in hospital, mother tired and anxious

estrogens (µg/24 hr)
regnanediol (mg/24 hr)

← Fertile-type mucus →

4.4
0.3

estrogens (µg/24 hr) 3.6 ... 4.4
regnanediol (mg/24 hr) 0.3 ... 0.3

Weaning complete

Wet

1 feed dropped
solids increased

9.6
0.2

I — 1 feed dropped, solids increased — 1 feed dropped

estrogen (µg/24 hr) 4.6
regnanediol (mg/24 hr) 0.2

Wet

5.8
0.3

← Wet, clear, slippery 20.8
0.3

17.6
0.3

5.4
2.4

6.8 O (µg/24 hr) 4.0
0.5 P (mg/24 hr) 0.4

— Cloudy mucus —

6.0
0.3

Clear Clear Wet

Wet
29.4
0.4

8.8
3.1

NOTE: I = Intercourse

Figure 7-7 (continued)

Return to Fertility in Nursing Mothers (continued)

I. Korea

1	2	3	4	5	6	7	8	9	10	11	12	13	14	15	16	17	18	19	20	21	22	23	24	25	26	27	28	29	30	31	32	33	34	3

J. United States

1	2	3	4	5	6	7	8	9	10	11	12	13	14	15	16	17	18	19	20	21	22	23	24	25	26	27	28	29	30	31	32	33	34	3

NOTE: I = Intercourse

K.

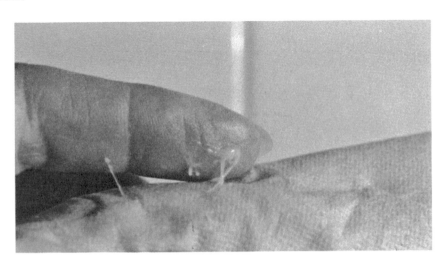

The chart shown in Figure 7–7F is that of an Australian woman who began charting 11 months after childbirth. The lochia had lasted for about 31 days, after which the woman was dry for seven months. She totally breast-fed her baby for five and one half months. Solid foods were then added to the baby's diet but no liquid supplements other than water. The woman's mucous secretion gradually reappeared. This chart is from the time when the baby was 12 months old, the woman returned to total breast-feeding when the family was vacationing. During those 17 days the mucous secretion was suppressed (see arrow in lines 1 and 2).

Laboratory studies showed that the appearance of clear, elastic mucus coincided with a significant increase in the woman's blood levels of estrogens (the days of the highest estrogen levels are indicated on the chart by heavy lines). The woman correctly predicted the return of menstruation from the date of her first ovulation after childbirth, as indicated on the chart (Line 11, column 1).

Note that a white baby stamp was used whenever the mucus changed from the basic infertile pattern (yellow stamp), a pattern that occurred without any change for several days at a time. The white baby stamp indicated that intercourse must be avoided while waiting for any possible change in the mucus. Intercourse must be avoided during the presence of any clear, elastic mucus until the fourth day after such mucus had disappeared or changed.

In the chart of the Indian woman (Figure 7–7G), note that the patches of mucus were similar during the weaning stages and then gradually returned to normal when weaning was completed.

The chart shown in Figure 7–7H is that of an Australian woman who began charting 3-1/2 months after childbirth. She and her husband wanted to avoid pregnancy, and they had abstained from intercourse since the birth.

She had not previously followed the Ovulation Method. From her chart you can see that she had a basic infertile pattern of dryness and one of slight sticky mucus. The couple was asked to follow the early days rule and place a white baby stamp the day after intercourse in case seminal fluid and the constant infertile mucus discharge would disguise the appearance of the beginning of the ovulatory phase. Observe that on the fifth line some bleeding was recorded, accompanied by fertile type mucus. This coincided with the time she had her children sick in the hospital and she was tired and anxious. As the number of feedings decreased and more solids were introduced, mucus of the fertile type appeared leading to ovulation. Hormonal measurements confirmed that ovulation had taken place (lines 9 and 11).

The chart shown in Figure 7–7I is that of a 33-year-old Korean woman, the mother of two children. Her baby, two years old, was still being breast-fed. Although the woman had observed cloudy, sticky mucus, she did not start charting until the baby was one year old, when clear, elastic mucus appeared. At one point (line 5), she had a continuous infectious discharge that was cured with medication. Note that for the first time in two years she observed clear, elastic mucus (line 5). After that, the luteal phase before her first menstrual period was fairly short. Perhaps that cycle was anovulatory, one in which the hormone levels were elevated enough to produce the mucous signs of ovulation but not elevated enough to produce ovulation itself. (Brown 1978).

The length of time between birth and the return of ovulation is different in different women. Eventually ovulation returns, even in the woman who is totally breast-feeding. Only rarely does it return in the first three months after birth. The chart shown in Figure 7–7J is that of an American woman, who, although she totally breast-fed her baby, menstruated within six weeks of delivery. Experienced in the Ovulation Method, she realized that fertility had returned even though she was nursing a big, hungry baby. She avoided intercourse during the days that mucus was present. The irregularity in the length of her cycles may have been due to the fact that she was still totally breast-feeding.

Another unusual condition that has been reported during breast-feeding is the prolonged secretion of clear, elastic mucus. It is the experience of teachers of the Ovulation Method that the secretion can be altered by adjusting the stimulation provided by the suckling. If suckling is increased by increased nursing, the clear, elastic secretion is reduced or it may totally disappear within a few days. If suckling is diminished, ovulation ensues.

The mucus that heralds the first ovulation after childbirth may not be as obviously fertile or infertile as it is at other times, probably because ovulation in the woman who is breast-feeding occurs under relatively low levels of estrogens (Brown 1978). If there is any indication that fertility may be returning, intercourse must not take place if pregnancy is to be avoided.

The time from the first ovulation and the following menstrual period can be relatively short. The first menstrual flow may be longer and more profuse, and the first few cycles may be irregular. Some women have a continuous milky mucous flow, that is their basic infertile pattern while they are breast-feeding. It is sometimes profuse and milky (Figure 7–7K). When normal cycles return the mucous pattern changes. The woman may have dry days after menstruation, then sticky, cloudy mucus, then milky, slippery mucus that resembles the mucus secreted while the woman was breast-feeding.

Women in developing countries, even those in the poorest and most primitive communities, space their children by breast-feeding for long periods of time. The protective elements in the mother's milk enable her infant to survive the conditions under which some people in those countries live. The women in those countries nurse

Figure 7–8. *A.* Irregular cycles in a 40-year-old woman. They may indicate the beginning of the premenopause. *B.* Irregular cycles and extensive intermittent bleeding with mucus. The woman disregarded the rules and became pregnant. *C.* Irregularities similar to those shown in *B.* But the woman followed the rules and avoided pregnancy. *D.* Irregular cycles and the absence of fertile mucous secretion may mean that the woman is premenopausal. *E.* Profuse bleeding and clotting are not uncommon during the premenopausal stage. Though illiterate, the woman was able to follow the rules and thus avoid pregnancy. *F.* Even if ovulation has taken place, conception does not occur if the right type of mucus necessary for the sperm to survive is not present. The numbers under the stamps refer to the hormonal correlations. O = total urinary estrogen (in micrograms/24 hr); P = urinary pregnanediol (in milligrams/24 hr).

Figure 7-8

Pre-Menopausal Women

A. United States

B. Canada

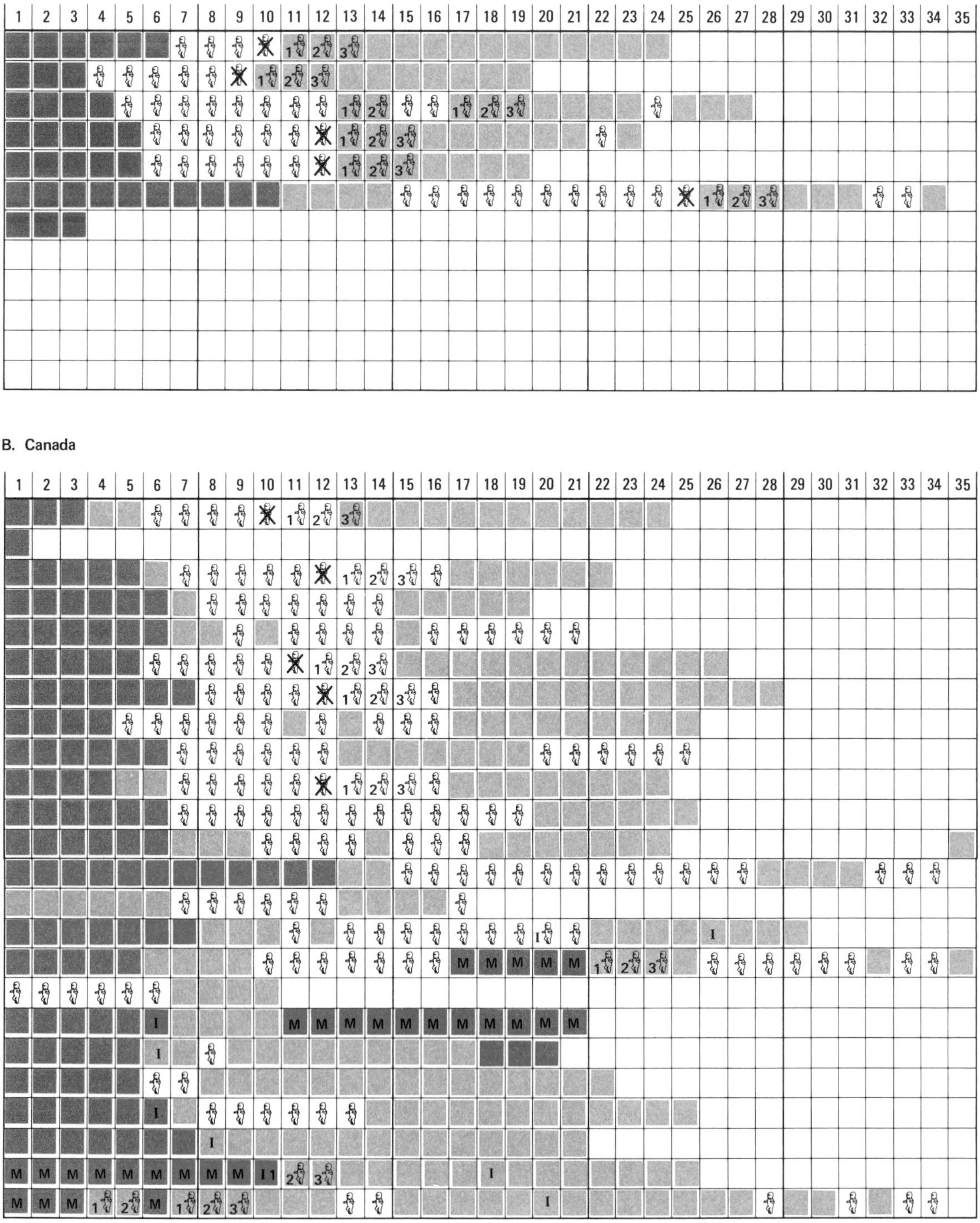

NOTE: I = Intercourse

Figure 7-8 (continued)   Pre-Menopausal Women (continued)

C. Australia

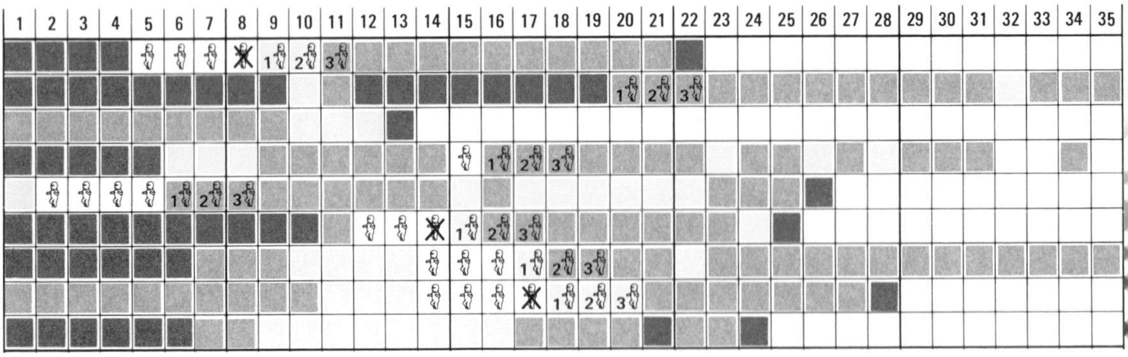

D. Fiji

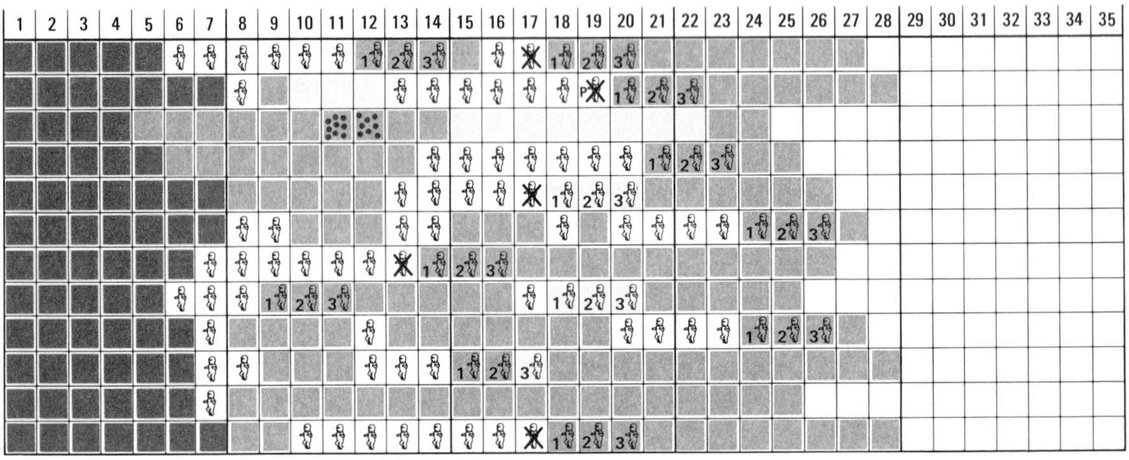

E. India

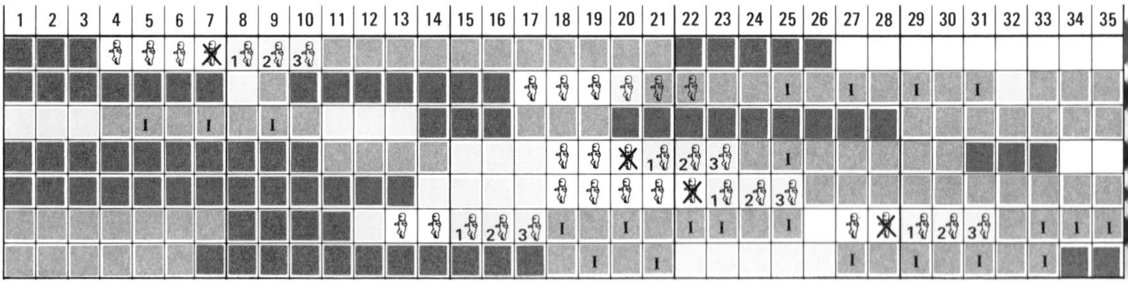

F. Australia

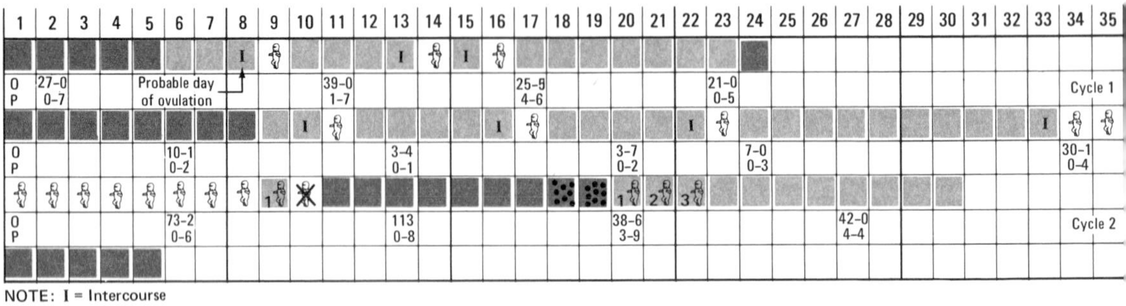

NOTE: I = Intercourse

their babies far more frequently than do women from more affluent societies, who for convenience or other reasons space the feedings further apart. Women in developing countries, who must care for their babies continously, carry them on their backs and nurse them frequently—on demand. The continued stimulation thus provided, delays the woman's return to fertility by blocking the hormonal messages that trigger ovulation.

OVULATION IN THE PREMENOPAUSAL WOMAN

The years during which a woman experiences a progressive decline in her fertility (usually when she is 45 to 55 years old) are referred to in this discussion as the premenopause.

During the premenopause, the menstrual periods may stop abruptly and begin again, or they may become very irregular, sometimes with profuse bleeding. Ovulation may occur only infrequently, or not at all, and even when menstruation is still occurring. In such a case, the woman could still be fertile. Fertile mucus may decline or disappear, in which case even a woman who is ovulating would be infertile (Figure 7-8F, page 90). Finally, the luteal phase of the cycle may become much shorter than the usual two weeks.

Besides the changes just mentioned, the woman may experience "hot flashes", in which a feeling of heat suffuses the body, and the face and neck get red. Hot flashes are a reflection of low estrogen levels (Billings 1976). (It may be of some consolation to the woman to know that the days on which she has hot flashes, she is infertile.) Women who are premenopausal are often depressed, perhaps because of the physical changes or from psychological reasons or both.

The premenopausal woman has changes in her mucous pattern. She may have many weeks of days on which she is dry or on which she has a continuous secretion of mucus that may be sticky or flaky. The continuous mucus in the premenopausal woman is composed of vaginal cells and white blood cells, and is a reflection of low estrogen levels (Billings 1976).

The charts shown in Figure 7-8 to illustrate charting during the premenopause are again those of women from different countries and cultures, to show that women everywhere have the same problems and are able to solve them using the Ovulation Method.

The chart shown in Figure 7-8A is that of a 45-year-old American woman who had had seven children. During her childbearing years, her cycles varied in length from 19 to 27 days. Cycle 6 was 34 days long for the first time in her life, and the increase in length might mean that the woman's premenopause stage is commencing.

The chart shown in Figure 7-8B is that of a 45-year-old woman whose cycles ranged in length from 19 to 28 days in the first year shown. In six of the cycles, ovulation may not have occurred since no clear, elastic mucus was observed. Yellow stamps, which were introduced some time after the chart shown here was made, could now be used instead of the white baby stamps in the apparently anovulatory cycles. In the second year, the woman's cycles were more irregular. Long cycles of cloudy, sticky mucus were followed by intermittent bleeding with mucus (line 4 and

6). Analysis of the days of intercourse in the second year shows that the couple disregarded the rule about avoiding intercourse during any day of bleeding (see page 89). The letter "M" marked on some of the red stamps indicated that mucus accompanied bleeding. In the next-to-last cycle, the woman had intercourse on the last day of bleeding, even though mucus and bleeding were present, and she became pregnant. It must be remembered that premenopausal women tend to have irregularities in the concentration of hormones that cause irregularities in the length of the cycles and also intermittent bleeding. Hence, the strict rules to avoid intercourse during the days of bleeding with mucus plus 3 days after.

tions seen in premenopausal women: (1) short fertile cycles—cycle 1, Line 1; (2) long cycles with intermittent bleeding—cycle 2, Lines 2 and 3; (3) anovulatory cycles— cycle 3, Lines 4 and 5; (4) prolonged bleeding—cycle 4, Line 6; (5) long fertile cycles —cycle 5, Lines 7 and 8; and (6) short, infertile cycles with only, dry flaky mucus— cycle 6, Line 9. In spite of the variations, the woman whose chart is shown avoided pregnancy by following the rules.

Similar variations are also shown in charts of women from developing countries and of different cultures See Figures 7–8D from Fiji and 7–8E from India. Note in the chart in Figure 7–8E the preponderance of irregular and apparently anovulatory cycles. According to her physician and her teacher of the Ovulation Method, the woman, a 39-year-old Hindu, had excessive bleeding and clotting. Such excessive bleeding is not uncommon during the premenopause. Even though the woman was illiterate, she was able to avoid pregnancy by following the rules. >Figure 7–8F belongs to a premenopausal mother from Australia. It is an excellent example that tells us that it is not always possible to know that ovulation has taken place in an individual cycle. But, it is possible to identify infertility by the characteristics of the type of mucus. The fact that a woman ovulates does not mean that she is capable of conceiving, unless the right type of fertile mucus necessary for the sperm to survive is present in the woman's body. In the first cycle the hormonal values seemed to indicate that ovulation had probably taken place on day 8. This day was dry and the act of intercourse did not result in conception. The white baby stamps placed each day after each act of intercourse indicate the presence of seminal fluid the day after intercourse. In the second cycle mucus with fertile characteristics was identified on the 45th day of the cycle Line 3. An X was placed then as bleeding occurred for nine days; three dry days of abstinence followed, a safe precaution in women approaching menopause, as both bleeding and a prolonged mucous secretion are common during the change of life. The hormonal measurements indicated that ovulation probably took place on the last day of bleeding. The appearance of mucus with some fertile characteristics just prior to the breakthrough bleed on the 45th day reflected the rise in ovarian estrogen levels which warned the woman of a possible approach of fertility.

Errata Sheet

The second paragraph on page 92 should read:

The chart in Figure 7-8C, that of an Australian woman, shows many of the variations seen in premenopausal women: (1) short fertile cycles — cycle 1, Line 1; (2) long cycles with intermittent bleeding — cycle 2, Lines 2 and 3; (3) anovulatory cycles — cycle 3, Lines 4 and 5; (4) prolonged bleeding — cycle 4, Line 6; (5) long fertile cycles — cycle 5, Lines 7 and 8; and (6) short, infertile cycles with only dry, flaky mucus — cycle 6, Line 9. In spite of the variations, the woman whose chart is shown avoided pregnancy by following the rules.

Pages 188–194 are reprinted with permission from *Hospital Progress,* August 1978. Copyright 1978 by The Catholic Health Association.

Therefore, women undergoing the premenopause should keep in mind that bleeding and an extended period of time of mucous discharge are fairly common at this stage of their life.

REFERENCES

Billings, E.L. *The Regulation of Births by the Ovulation Method at the Climacteric* (Change of Life). Natural Family Planning Council of Victoria, June, 1976.

8

Charting the Mucous Secretion After Discontinuance of the Pill and Other Artificial Contraceptives

Chapter 8 discusses the Pill, the intrauterine devices, and the injectable contraceptive. The discussion is limited to these particular contraceptives because they are the ones most commonly used, and many women who are learning the Ovulation Method have recently used one of those methods. Thus, it is important that teachers of the Ovulation Method, and present and prospective users of the Ovulation Method, understand how these artificial methods of contraception work and what side effects are encountered, particularly those side effects that may be detrimental to a woman's health and fertility.

THE PILL

The many different types of oral contraceptives (all referred to in this book as the Pill) are composed of various combinations of synthetic and natural steroids that inhibit ovulation and/or the implantation of a fertilized ovum (Ayd, 1964). They also make the mucous secretion dense so that sperm are not able to penetrate it and reach the ovum (Hilgers, 1978, Hume, 1978). Hume and others think that the Pill sometimes works as an abortifacient, causing a fertilized ovum to be destroyed or rendering the uterine lining unfit to support implantation of a fertilized ovum.

SIDE EFFECTS OF THE PILL

The side effects of the Pill, the IUD and the injectable contraceptive, are being investigated—and argued about—with great intensity. The side effects discussed here and in other parts of the chapter range from those uncovered in what many consider definitive studies, to those that have been uncovered in research that is not yet completed. Whatever the stage of the research, women who are choosing a method of avoiding pregnancy should be aware that there is an effective method that presents no hazard to their physical health (the Ovulation Method), as well as other methods that may have an enormous number of dangerous side effects.

The list of possible side effects of the Pill given in the *Physician's Desk Reference*, and also inserted with the packages of the Pill, is a long one. The list includes edema, breakthrough bleeding, mental depression, and decrease in glucose tolerance, diabetes, thrombophlebitis, pulmonary embolism, cerebral vascular anomalies, and hepatomas and other disorders of the liver (see also Seaman and Seaman, 1977). There is also speculation among some scientists that prolonged use of the Pill could ultimately disturb the functioning of the brain, pituitary, ovaries, adrenal glands, liver, and uterus (*British Medical Journal,* 1977).

The Pill induces a pseudopregnant condition that some consider a pathological state in that the changes that occur, although appropriate to pregnancy, are irrelevant to the nonpregnant state and may thus favor the development of dangerous conditions, such as thrombosis and thromboembolism (FDA, 1978). A study of women in the United Kingdom taking the Pill showed that the death rate from a variety of causes was approximately five times greater in those women than in women who had never taken the Pill (Royal College of General Practitioners' Oral Contraception Study, *The Lancet,* 1977).

Amenorrhea, a common side effect of the Pill, may sometimes be long term. Although the amenorrhea is seldom permanent, the outlook for a successful pregnancy is "less rosy" (*British Medical Journal,* 1976). Some women who have discontinued the Pill because they wish to become pregnant may have more trouble than they anticipated since they are not menstruating.

Use of the Pill during pregnancy may increase the chances that the baby may be born with some defect, such as improper development of the limbs, or vertebral, cardiac, tracheal, esophageal, or genital anomalies (Hume, 1978; Seaman and Seaman, 1977).

Women taking the Pill may have vitamin B_6 and other types of nutritional deficiencies (Rose, 1966; Martinez and Roe, 1977). Seaman and Seaman also feel that use of the Pill may be related to the development of eye disorders, high blood pressure, diabetes, gall bladder trouble, decreased resistance to viral infections, and even cancer. In 1977 Stern and his coworkers reported an increasing possibility of cancer of the cervix in certain women who were taking the Pill. They based their projection on their five-year study of women who displayed an abnormality of the lining of the cervix that is known as dysplasia. Although an increased incidence of cervical cancer in Pill users is a matter of controversy, Stern's evidence indicates that prolonged use of the Pill increases the risk of cancer in women with dysplasia.

The Pill is an extraordinarily potent drug that affects a large number of body processes.

Charting the Mucous Secretion After Discontinuing the Pill

Women who begin to chart after discontinuing the Pill seem to show irregularities in their cycles, therefore they are warned by the Ovulation Method teacher that they should wait at least three to six months before attempting to become pregnant.

The charts shown in the following pages illustrate the various reactions women around the world have reported after they discontinued the Pill.

The chart shown in Figure 8–1A is that of an American woman who had discontinued the Pill after taking it for less than a year. The initial bleeding that followed was a "withdrawal" bleeding, not a true menstruation (page 95). After the initial bleeding, the woman had a prolonged mucous discharge. Such a discharge is common when a woman has been taking the Pill for a long period of time. As explained on page 5, ovulation occurs only when hormones have reached a certain level. Patches of infertile mucus occur when the levels are not high enough.

Note (in Figure 8–1A) that from the second cycle on, the cycles were normal and seemed fertile. The letter "M" at the bottom of the green stamps a few days before their menstrual period indicates the slight brownish mucus that many women have just before menstruation (page 50). Because the woman had been on the Pill for a relatively short time, she had no trouble following the Ovulation Method. But the records of women who have discontinued the Pill after many years on it are often more complicated.

The chart shown in Figure 8–1B is that of a young American woman. After taking the Pill for only eight months, the woman decided to discontinue it because it had affected her eyes. (She had also decided to become pregnant.) After charting for some months, she did not observe any mucus, except for a few patches of cloudy, sticky mucus. It took her a year and a half to become pregnant. (Several other cases of prolonged dryness and infertility after discontinuance of the Pill have been reported from different parts of the world.)

The chart shown in Figure 8–1C is that of a young Australian woman. After charting for some months, she was advised by her physician to take the Pill because she had severe menstrual cramps and she was expecting her menstrual period around the time of her wedding. She took two 21-day courses of the Pill, starting on the fifth day of the seventh cycle, right after her menstrual period. After this short exposure to the Pill she found that she was no longer able to recognize a Peak day, because her mucous discharge had changed considerably. She had intermittent discharges of slippery, stretchy, threadlike mucus. Although her early safe days were not completely dry, she was able to identify them by the continuous, unchanging character of the mucus. It took 6 cycles for her to return to normal even though she had taken only two 21-day courses of the Pill.

In the first normal cycle recorded after taking the pill on that same chart, line 13 the couple had intercourse on day 11 of a 27-day cycle (the entire luteal phase was 13 days) without becoming pregnant. In the last cycle, she had intercourse on day 10

Figure 8–1. After discontinuing the Pill. *A*. A long patch of sometimes fertile mucus is often observed. *B*. Occasionally a woman has no mucous secretion. The woman wanted to conceive, but she had to wait 18 months for her fertility to return. *C*. Although she took the pill for only one month (cycle 7), the woman's mucus pattern was disrupted for five cycles. She achieved pregnancy in the last cycle. *D*. Typical result of long use of the pill. Long periods of infertile mucous secretion and other irregularities. *E*. Short exposure to the Pill often has long-term effects, especially in women in developing countries. *F*. High blood pressure is one side effect of the Pill. The woman had taken the Pill for eight years. Hormone studies indicated that she was still infertile two years after discontinuation of the pill.

After Discontinuation of the Pill

Figure 8–1

A. United States

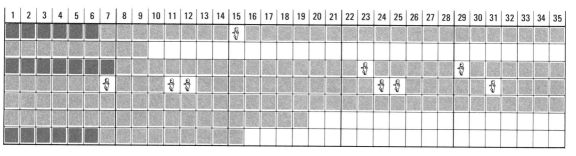

B. United States

C. Australia

NOTE: I = Intercourse

Figure 8-1 (continued)   After Discontinuation of the Pill (continued)

D. Canada

E. Dominican Republic

NOTE: **I** = Intercourse

F. Australia

1	2	3	4	5	6	7	8	9	10	11	12	13	14	15	16	17	18	19	20	21	22	23	24	25	26	27	28	29	30	31	32	33	34	35

NOTE: I = Intercourse

(the Peak day was day 16) and on day 20, and she became pregnant. At first it appeared that the method had failed (the woman had not planned to become pregnant), but later she and her husband said that they had had intimate genital contact around the Peak Day, not realizing that such contact could result in pregnancy (page 33).

The chart shown in Figure 8–1D is that of a Canadian woman who had been taking the Pill for many years. She had intermittent bleeding between cycles, as well as mucous discharges at different times in the cycle. Wanting to become pregnant, she had intercourse on days of possible fertility without success. She would have been wise, however, to allow her body time to return to its pre-Pill state before attempting to become pregnant, in view of the remote possibility of infant malformation. Furthermore, women who become pregnant soon after they have discontinued the Pill often have miscarriages.

The chart shown in Figure 8–1E is that of a woman from the Dominican Republic who had a severe response to a short exposure to the Pill. Such a severe reaction is not unusual in women from developing countries who often have poor diets and difficult living conditions. The woman had taken the Pill for only a few months. When she suspended the medication and began charting, she had an increase in cloudy, sticky mucus in the first cycle, and she had only cloudy, sticky mucus in the following cycles. Even though the mucus occurred at the time that ovulation might have been expected to occur, there was a poor mucous build-up and no clear, elastic mucus. Thus the woman did not seem to be ovulating normally. Obviously fertile before using the Pill (she had seven children), she seemed to be temporarily infertile after only a few months on the Pill.

The chart shown in Figure 8–1F is that of an Australian woman who began taking the Pill when she was in her midthirties. She took it for eight years, and she developed high blood pressure. After discontinuing the Pill, she began to use the Ovulation Method. Note that she has a continuous infertile mucous discharge as indicated by her yellow stamps. She also used yellow baby stamps throughout the chart to indicate the presence of seminal fluid on the days following intercourse. Hormone studies that continued through the second year verified that she had not yet begun ovulating.

Summary

The charts just discussed confirm what is known from research—that the Pill can continue to affect a woman's mucous secretion and ovulation for months after she has stopped taking it. In some women, exposure to the Pill as short as one month led to apparently anovulatory phases of as long as eight months. Other reactions to the Pill included a continuous mucous secretion, perhaps caused by a vaginal infection, and bleeding between cycles. Brown (1978) found low levels of urinary estrogen in women suffering from amenorrhea of various causes. Such low levels of estrogen indicate a lack of ovarian function. Users of the Pill expect to have signs of suppressed ovulation, but many former users of the Pill are surprised, and dismayed, to discover that the signs of suppressed ovulation may continue for weeks or months after the Pill has been discontinued. In some apparently anovulatory women, estrogen levels may rise or remain high, without a rise in pregnanediol. However, bleeding may occur because of the decrease in estrogen (Brown, 1978). Thus the normal increases and decreases in estrogen and progesterone are disturbed both while the woman is taking the Pill and after she has stopped taking it.

INTRAUTERINE DEVICES

Unlike the Pill, the several types of intrauterine devices (IUDs) do not suppress ovulation. Although it is not known exactly how the IUD acts, it is known that it works in the postovulatory phase of the cycle and that its activity centers on disturbing the implantation of a fertilized ovum. An IUD affects only the uterus, making it incapable of receiving and/or sustaining a fertilized ovum (Martin and Brown, 1973). Thus the IUD seems to act as an abortifacient (Hilgers, 1974). In many women, the luteal phase of the cycle is shortened after the insertion of an IUD. An IUD alters the lining of the uterus and the underlying layer of muscle. In women not using an IUD, muscular activity in the uterus is normally diminished after ovulation, but in women who have an IUD in place, uterine contractions that have been likened to those in the early stages of labor begin four or five days after ovulation (Bengtsson and Moawad, 1967). The increased muscular activity occurs about the time that implantation of a fertilized ovum would occur if the woman had become pregnant.

Side Effects of the IUD

Many people do not realize that the use of an IUD has its dangers. The IUD may cause injury while it is being inserted, while it remains in place, and when it is being removed. Reports from developing countries state that the uterus is often perforated during the removal because the paramedic removing it has not had sufficient training and experience. Perforation of the uterus during removal of an IUD occurs in highly developed countries also (Seaman and Seaman, 1977). Some IUDs are so designed that they are easier to insert than to remove. The uterus, in an effort to reject the foreign device, sets up a continuous irritation that is often accompanied by infection.

According to Seaman and Seaman, "pathologists who have studied the changes in the uterus caused by the IUD generally loathe it and have consistently warned against it. Many family planners are unaware of these studies or are indifferent to them."

Charting After Removal of an IUD

Figure 8–2 shows the charts of women who began to use the Ovulation Method after removal of an IUD. The charts show the various conditions that can result from use of the IUD. If an infectious discharge is not present when the IUD is removed, the mucous pattern is normal, as can be seen in Figure 8–2A (cycles 1 to 4). The woman wanted to become pregnant. In the fifth cycle, she had intercourse during the fertile days, and she conceived.

The chart shown in Figure 8–2B is that of a Mexican American woman, the mother of five children. She started charting while she still had the IUD in place because she wanted to observe any mucous discharge. With the IUD in place, she had many more days of mucous secretion than she had otherwise. The constant state of inflammation induced by the IUD probably caused the increase in the mucus. In the cycle immediately after the removal of the IUD, the woman did not have a Peak day (line 4). She had intercourse on the fifteenth day of that cycle, just before a small build-up of cloudy, sticky mucus. The subsequent cycles were perfectly normal.

The chart shown in Figure 8–2C is that of an American woman who had an almost continuous discharge after removal of an IUD. She was still able to pinpoint her fertile phase accurately. Because the discharge persisted, her doctor treated her for cervicitis, cauterizing her cervix. She then had an increased discharge of cloudy, sticky mucus, but she was able to distinguish that from the clear, elastic mucus. The woman commented that the two types of discharge remained separate, like oil and water, a phenomenon that enabled her to distinguish them easily.

After removal of the IUD, women can expect an average of a one to three month interval before returning to normal cycles, unless there is a severe infection. Thus, the IUD, like the Pill, may disrupt cyclicity after its removal, but its effects seem less severe in this respect than those of the Pill.

INJECTABLE CONTRACEPTIVES

Depo-Provera (depo medroxyprogesterone acetate) is the most popular of the injectable contraceptives (Population Reports, 1975). In 1975, Depo-Provera (D-P) was available for use in over 64 countries. It is estimated that over one million women now use injectable progesterones for contraceptive purposes. Some of the advantages cited for D-P are that it is highly effective in preventing pregnancy, on a par with oral contraceptives; it is easy to administer and long lasting (one injection lasts from three to six months), it is popular in developing countries, where injections are associated with modern medical techniques; and it is safe to administer to nursing mothers. The last point is debatable, however, since D-P and (or) its metabolic by-products can be found in the breast milk of women on D-P. Long-range studies of its effect on infants have not been done. The disadvantages of D-P are that it disturbs menstrual patterns while it is being used; it may shorten or lengthen the cycle and often causes amenorrhea; it cannot be withdrawn if problems arise; and after long-term use a delay in return of fertility and cyclicity may be experienced. After two years of D-P use, 40 per cent of the women may be amenorrheic. The median time to return to fertility is 13 months and ranges up to three years.

Figure 8-2. *A*. After five cycles in which there were normal mucous secretions, the woman had intercourse around the Peak day, and she became pregnant. *B*. An IUD was removed during the woman's third cycle. After one cycle in which there was no fertile mucus, she had normal cycles. *C*. After removal of the IUD, the woman had a continuous mucous discharge. Although her cervix was cauterized in the second cycle, she was able to distinguish fertile from infertile mucus.

Figure 8-3. *A*. After cessation of the Depo-Provera, the woman had heavy bleeding. She returned to normal in four months. *B*. After cessation of the Depo-Provera, the woman continued to bleed. *C*. Irregularity after only one three-month injection. The irregularity may have been aggravated by her poor diet. *D*. After four injections of Depo-Provera, the woman was irregular and she probably was not ovulating. Fertile mucus did not appear until cycle 7 (line 10).

Figure 8–2

After Removal of an IUD

United States

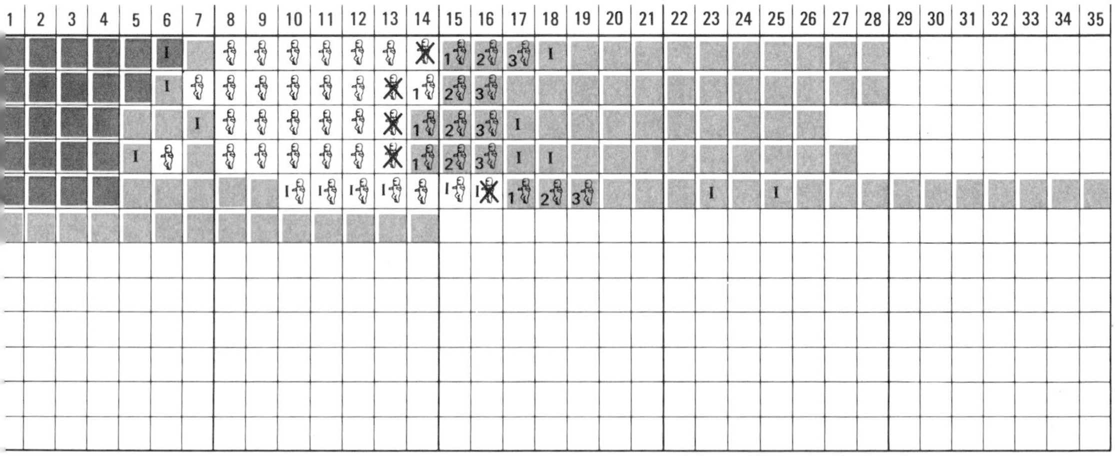

1	2	3	4	5	6	7	8	9	10	11	12	13	14	15	16	17	18	19	20	21	22	23	24	25	26	27	28	29	30	31	32	33	34	35

Mexico

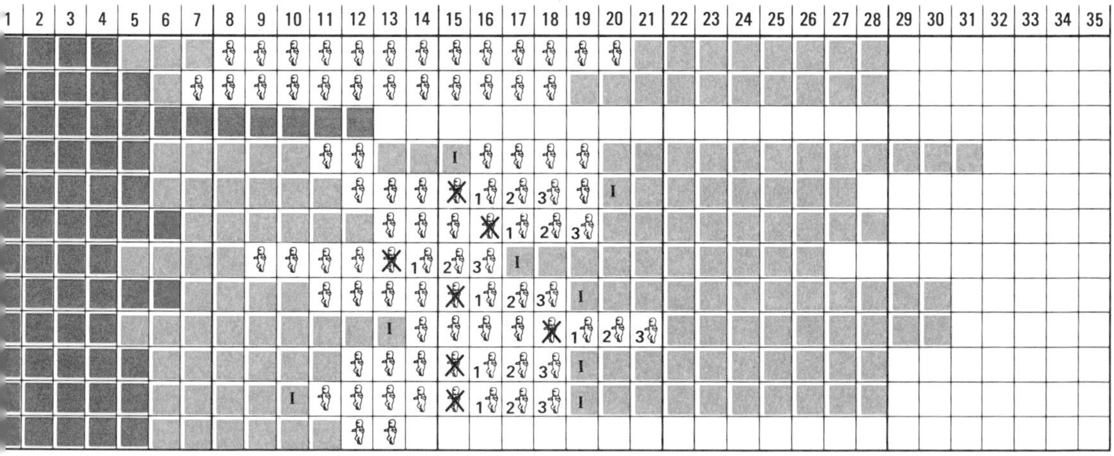

1	2	3	4	5	6	7	8	9	10	11	12	13	14	15	16	17	18	19	20	21	22	23	24	25	26	27	28	29	30	31	32	33	34	35

United States

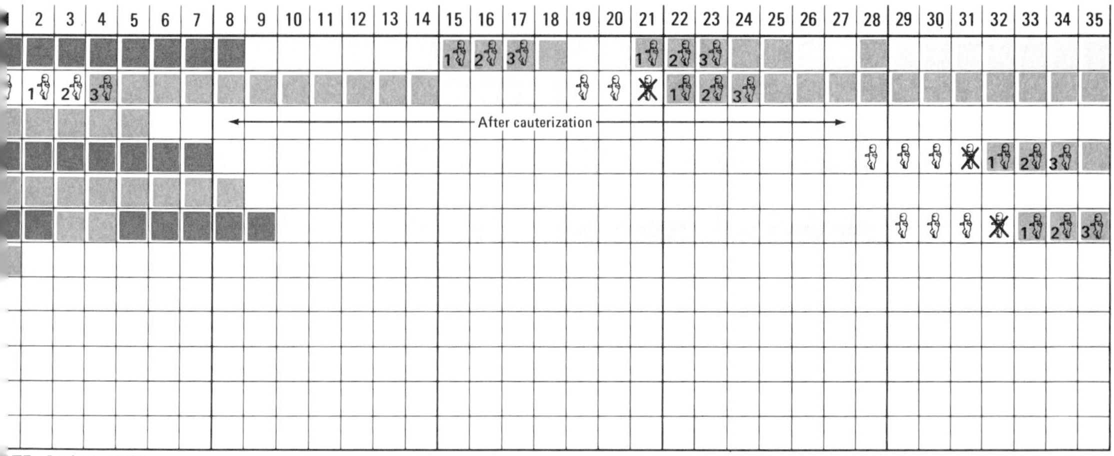

	2	3	4	5	6	7	8	9	10	11	12	13	14	15	16	17	18	19	20	21	22	23	24	25	26	27	28	29	30	31	32	33	34	35

After cauterization

NOTE: I = Intercourse

Figure 8-3

After Discontinuation of Depo-Provera

A. Mexico

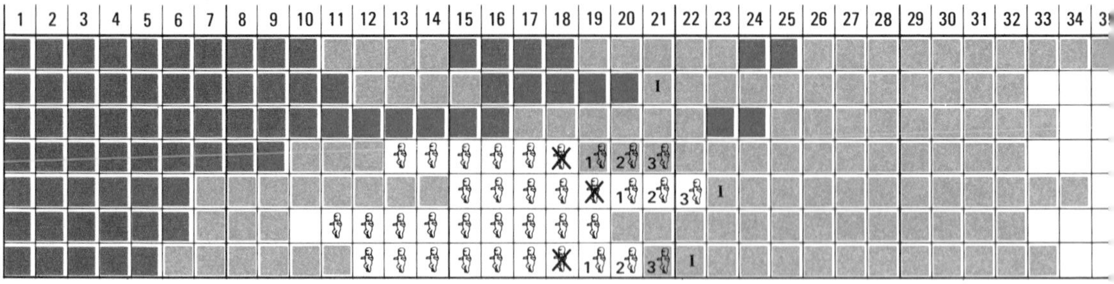

B. Mexico

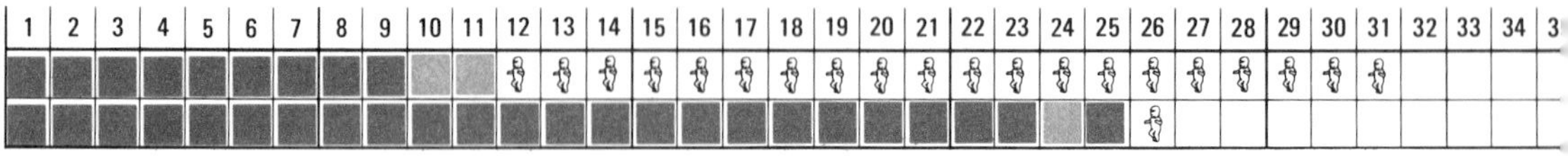

C. Fiji

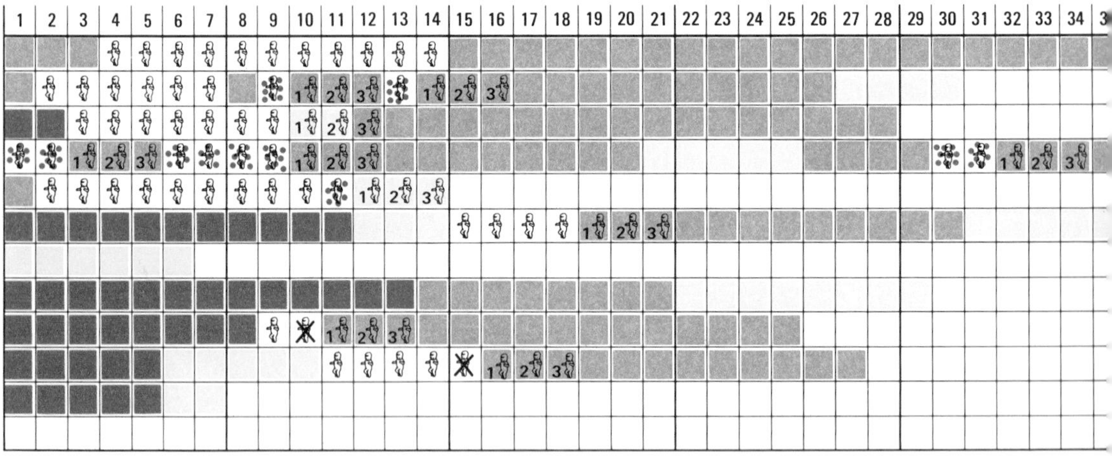

D. Fiji

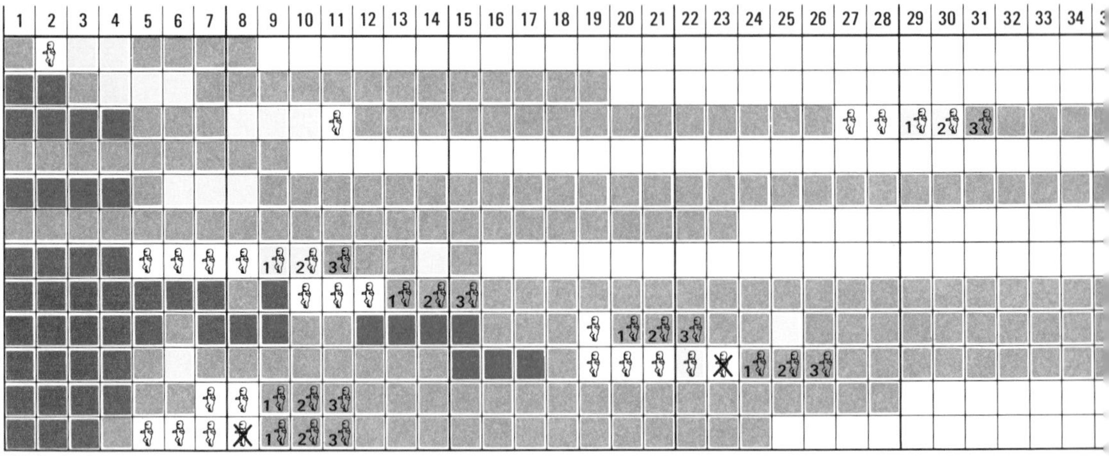

NOTE: I = Intercourse

D-P has a long history of use and/or abuse. Because of fears about the long-term effects of D-P, especially the danger of permanent infertility, the Food and Drug Administration did not approve its use as a contraceptive. Currently, the only approved use of D-P in the United States is for treatment of advanced endometrial cancer. The irregular and excessive bleeding patterns experienced by D-P users are often treated by administering oral estrogens. That, in effect, eliminates one of the advantages of D-P, in that the daily treatment makes it similar to being on oral contraceptives. Other problems that occur as side effects in D-P users are weight gain, increase in blood glucose levels, nausea, dizziness, headaches, acne, nervousness and painful menstruation. There is also debate over cancer risks in D-P users. Some statistics suggest that cervical carcinoma occurs more frequently in D-P users. Additionally, animal research has implicated D-P in producing breast nodules; human studies, however, do not report a correlation between D-P and breast nodules.

D-P, like other hormonal contraceptives, such as the Pill, works by inhibiting ovulation, by changing the uterine endometrial lining, and by changing the viscosity of the cervical mucus. In essence, it eliminates fertility at each possible stage. It blocks ovulation, but if ovulation were to occur implantation would be unlikely. Finally, D-P alters the mucus so that it becomes impenetrable to sperm.

Charting the Mucous Secretion After Discontinuing Depo-Provera

Figure 8–3 shows the charts of women from Mexico and Fiji who had been using the contraceptive injection. After discontinuing it, they had severe hemorrhages that would have aggravated any anemia that women with such poor diets were likely to have.

Figure 8–3A belongs to a 35 year old illiterate Mexican woman, mother of five, who used the injection for a year. Severe side effects forced her to discontinue, and severe bleeding occurred for the following three months, see lines 1, 2 and 3.

Figure 8–3B shows the chart of a 30-year-old woman from Mexico, the mother of six children. She used the contraceptive injection for 1-1/2 years. After discontinuing it, she also had continuous bleeding for a long period of time.

The chart shown in Figure 8–3C is that of a 39-year-old woman from Fiji, the mother of four children. She had only one injection, given six weeks after the delivery of her last child. The great irregularity of her cycles may have been caused by her poor diet, as well as by the injection. She had intermittent bleeding between cycles, profuse bleeding during her menstrual periods, and an almost continuous mucous discharge. Introduced to the yellow stamps when she began to chart, she was able to distinguish the infertile discharge from her fertile mucus. Thus she was able to use the Ovulation Method without difficulty. Her last cycle indicated a possible return to normalcy.

The chart shown in Figure 8–3D is that of a 28-year-old woman from Fiji, the mother of four children. She was given her first contraceptive injection when her youngest baby was six weeks old and her last injection when the baby was 10 months old. Altogether, she received four injections. Her diet was good, consisting of dalo, tapioca, meat, and leafy vegetables. Her first six cycles were apparently anovulatory and of varying lengths. In the seventh cycle (line 10), she had clear, elastic mucus for the first time since she had discontinued the injection.

REFERENCES

Ayd, Frank. *"The Oral Contraceptive." Medical Newsletter for Religious.* 1964. Baltimore, Maryland.

Bengtsson, L.P., and Moawad, A.H., *Am. J. of Obstetrics and Gynaecology* **98**: 957, (1967).

British Medical Journal, An editorial, "Amenorrhoea after Oral Contraceptives," 1976, **2**, 660–661.

British Medical Journal, An editorial, 1977. **2**: 918.

Brown, J.B. "Hormonal Correlations of the Ovulation Method." Paper presented at the *International Conference on the Ovulation Method,* 1978. Melbourne, Australia.

Food and Drug Administration (FDA) USA. "Detailed Patient Labelling," 1978. Washington, DC.

Hilgers, Thomas. "The Pill and the IUD, Contraceptive or Abortifacient?" Minnesota *Medical.* June, 1974. **57**: 493–501.

Hume, Kevin. "Physical Consequences of Contraception: The Metabolic Mischief of the Pill." Paper presented at *International Conference, Humanae Vitae,* 1978, Melbourne, Australia.

Martin, Peter, and Brown, James. "The Effect of Intrauterine Contraceptive Devices on Ovarian and Menstrual Function in the Human." *Journal of Clinical Endocrinology Metabolism,* 1973, **36**. 1125–1131.

Martinez, Olga and Roe, Daphne. "Effect of Oral Contraceptives on Blood Folate Levels in Pregnancy." *American Journal of Obstetrics and Gynecology,* 1977, **128**, 255–261.

Physician's Desk Reference, 30th Edition, 1976. Oradell, N.J.: Medical Economics Co.

Population Reports. "Injectables and Implants." Department of Medical and Public Affairs, The George Washington University Medical Center, Washington, DC, 1975.

Rose, D.P. "Apparent Vitamin B_6 Deficiency Induced by the Ingestion of Oral Contraceptives." *Nature,* 1966, **210**, 197.

Royal College of General Practitioners' Oral Contraception Study, "Mortality Among Oral-Contraceptive Users," *The Lancet,* 1977, **2,** 727–731.

Seaman, Barbara and Seaman, Gideon. *Women and the Crisis in Sex Hormones.* New York: Rawson Associates Publishers, Inc., 1977.

Stern, Elizabeth, Forsythe, Alan, Youkeles, Lee and Coffelt, Carl. "Steroid Contraceptive Use and Cervical Dysplasia: Increased Risk of Progression." *Science,* 1977, **196**, 1460–1462.

9

Teaching the Ovulation Method to Teenagers and Young Adults

The comments in this chapter are directed to all those people who play a role in the education of young people in regard to sexuality—parents, teachers, counselors, and administrators of the various sex education programs. Since basic anatomy and physiology of reproduction have been covered elsewhere (pages 3–23), this chapter addresses itself to other considerations in sex education, including attitudes toward sexuality and the responsibility human beings have for safeguarding their procreative powers.

Parents are the first and most important teachers of sexuality since through exposure to the parents the child develops his/her unconscious ideas about sexuality and about himself/herself as a sexual person. Ideally, the parents are also the best ones to instruct the child formally in sex education since they are in a position to be sensitive to the individual needs of their children. Unfortunately, many parents are, for one reason or another, reluctant to undertake their children's sex education, and the task is delegated to others.

Whether the sex instruction is given in the home or in school, the scientific information should be given in conjunction with attitudes toward reproduction. People of all ages are capable of acting maturely and responsibly in their sexual activities as in other aspects of their lives. Young people have shown themselves determined and disciplined in working toward many different goals. There is no reason to expect that young people are not able to use their sexual energies responsibly. Those adults who push young people into sexual activity on the grounds that sexual urges cannot be resisted are treating young people condescendingly.

In recent years people of all ages have become intensely interested in learning about the body and how to keep it fit. And it is only natural that there should be an especially deep interest in learning about reproductive capacities since the physical integrity of the human race depends on their functioning. The reproductive system is at least as complicated as any other body system. Young people (and others) are fascinated to find out that the brain controls the functioning of the reproductive organs. After having discussed that fact, the teacher can go on to explain the complex interactions of the brain, pituitary gland, and the ovaries that result in ovulation (pages 3–8).

A discussion of the harmonious functioning of the reproductive organs often prompts young people to ask about the chemical and physical mechanisms involved in the use of artificial contraceptives. After it is certain that the young people understand the fundamentals of the interaction of the reproductive organs, they are asked to visualize their organs working together as do the parts of a finely tuned machine. In every normal menstrual cycle, all the organs work together in the appropriate way and at the appropriate time to prepare an incubation medium in the uterus that can support and nourish a developing baby. If fertilization and implantation do not occur, the body is directed to discharge the nourishing lining of the uterus, and menstruation occurs.

The teacher then explains how the various artificial birth control devices interfere with that synchrony of events and the functions of each organ. The contraceptive pills on the market act by inhibiting ovulation or as is now being suspected, the low dose Pill may affect implantation of a fertilized ovum (Hilgers, 1977; Ratner, 1978). Thus a functional abortion may occur, and in addition to its contraceptive and/or abortifacient effects, the Pill affects each organ controlling reproduction, as well as other organs (pages 95–100).

Young people are astonished to learn that a product with so many and such highly questionable results is so widely used. They are surprised that science is not more precise and responsible in its diversion of a normal bodily function. The warning listed by the FDA (1978) that use of the pill during adolescence may temporarily or permanently alter the biological systems involved in reproduction (page 95) is even more alarming.

Other methods, such as the intrauterine device (IUD) are not free of some dangerous side effects (refer to Chapter 8). An IUD in place protrudes a nylon thread into the upper vagina. The thread is a convenient ladder by which bacteria can penetrate to the uterine cavity, particularly during ovulation and menstruation, when the cervix opens. Wearers of the IUD report heavy menstrual bleeding and unplanned pregnancies. Nurses often describe cases in which babies have been delivered with an IUD attached to their bodies.

Abortion is used as a last-ditch method of birth control, even for young girls and without parental consent. It is estimated that one million abortions are performed every year in the United States.

Through the media, adolescents have been exposed to arguments for and against abortion, and the teacher probably does not need to review them. The film *Abortion— A Woman's Decision* (Acta Films, Chicago, Ill.) gives information on abortion at various stages of pregnancy that is new to most viewers. Boys as well as girls have a right to know all the facts about abortion. Too often the rights and responsibility of the man have been overlooked when abortion is being considered. The incidence of veneral disease has risen sharply during the past decade. Gonorrhea is particularly treacherous to women because it usually has no symptoms until complications become apparent. By that time, the fallopian tubes may have become infected or blocked with scar tissue which can result in permanent sterility.

In teaching sex education to young people (and older people), it should not be assumed that those being instructed know even the basics of reproduction. Certain facts seem always to come as a surprise—that a girl is born with the total number of eggs in her ovaries that she will have for her entire reproductive life, and that a boy manufactures spermatozoa continuously from the time of puberty. It is also not generally known that girls do not usually begin to ovulate until about two years after menstruation first begins (Brown 1978).

Instruction should be given also about other aspects of reproduction—childbirth, breast-feeding, natural family planning, menopause, and so on. Much of the anxiety and uncertainty connected with childbirth could be reduced by more knowledge. For example, many women trying to decide whether or not to breast-feed their babies do not know that nursing brings physical and emotional benefits to the mother as well as to the child. Data indicate that women who receive the proper instruction and support (as through the La Leche League, for example) usually decide to breast-feed their children (page 88).

Perhaps the lessons learned by teenagers who have had easy access to contraception and unlimited sexual license will bring about a countertrend towards responsible sexual behavior.

A poll was taken in 1977 of 24,000 juniors and seniors chosen to be listed in *Who's Who Among American High School Students*. Although seven out of 10 students said they did not condemn couples' living together without marriage, only two of the seven said that they would consider such a relationship for themselves.

Seventy percent of high school students questioned said that they had never had sexual intercourse. Fifty-six percent said that they would prefer their husband or wife to be a virgin at the time of marriage. Morality, not parental pressure or lack of opportunity, was given as the chief reason. A poll taken a few years earlier indicated a much higher rate of promiscuity.

I would like to quote excerpts from a letter of Dr. John Brennan to the Secretary of Health, Education and Welfare, which I feel summarizes the most important points regarding responsible sex education to the young.

"Of far greater value to the health care of our teenagers would be your leadership role in a national program to protect their inner reproductive organs by the most effective and least expensive form of birth control, sexual abstinence.

"Along with the rights of reproductive freedom comes responsibility and with responsibility come rewards.

1. Freedom from unwanted pregnancy
2. Freedom from complications of the pill and IUD
3. Freedom from venereal disease
4. Freedom from early sterilization from either V.D. or unwanted pregnancy
5. Freedom from complications of abortion
6. Freedom from forms of genital cancer
7. Freedom from the stigma and sorrow that befalls a family with an unmarried pregnant daughter
8. Freedom to explore cerebrocentric rather than genitocentric sexuality

"The need for self discipline in sexuality is no different from the need for that trait in every other aspect of our daily lives.

"Dr. John Billings of Australia has put the emphasis on ovulation. Teenagers should be taught that the thousand little eggs deep in the ovaries of young girls are their gift of life to be protected until the right environment is present to produce children.

"Nature has dictated that young people are physically able to reproduce as soon as they become teenagers. They must be taught that intelligence and self control are essential. Social, economic, and educational standards dictate that they must wait a time of perhaps ten years before it is to their advantage to reproduce. Total success in avoiding unwanted pregnancy, abortion, venereal disease, complications of the pill and the IUD depends not upon further advances in technology but upon a strong national program stressing the advantages of discipline.

"It would be a strange society indeed if the government said cigarettes are wrong, alcohol is wrong, drugs are wrong, lying, stealing, and all forms of violence are wrong, but in sex you can do no wrong.

"It is the job of parents and educators to assure young people that they are capable of leading ordered and responsible sexual lives, propaganda to the contrary not withstanding. Everyone has a responsibility to his own body, to the welfare of those he loves and is responsible for, and to society at large, including the generations to come."

REFERENCES

Brennan, J. Letter to Secretary of HEW, 1978.
Brown, J. B. "Hormonal Correlations of the Ovulation Method." Paper presented at the International Conference on the Ovulation Method, Melbourne, Australia, 1978.
Hilgers, Thomas. St. John's Conference, 1977.
Kane, Lawrence J. Personal communication, 1977.
Ratner, H. Personal communication, 1978.

10

Teaching the Ovulation Method in Developing Countries

The Ovulation Method has been successfully taught in developing countries. This chapter describes some of the approaches used in these countries, as well as some of the problems connected with the instruction.

Whatever the culture, the teacher must be careful to approach the people with respect for their way of life including their religious practices. Teachers know from experience that every woman who is determined to learn the Method can learn it, and thus the teacher encourages the learner to expect success.

CULTURAL DIFFERENCES

In one center in Guatemala the first class is devoted to a discussion of how difficult it is for Guatemalans to talk about sex. The discussion that ensues is usually a long one, with the people finally agreeing that they need to learn. The teacher also tactfully reminds the people that since their children are sometimes attaining higher levels of education than their parents, they are becoming more sophisticated about sexual matters, but are afraid to discuss sex in their homes because *costumbre* (custom) forbids it.

In Papua New Guinea, it is easy to teach and learn the Ovulation Method, because the women have only two or three days of mucus, and, finally, only dry days until the next menstruation. In a really primitive village, where the nutrition is poor, a woman might have only one day of mucus with fertile characteristics.

Each geographical area in Papua New Guinea has its own word for mucus, and possibly only the women know the word. When the woman moves to an urban area, where the nutrition may be better, the number of days of mucous secretion may well increase (see page 54).

In Moresby, many women are learning the Ovulation Method so that they can become pregnant. The charts of these women show green (dry) days all the time. Interestingly, if these women are given vitamin E, often the mucous secretion starts. The association of mucus increase and vitamin E has only recently been observed (Adrian 1978), and only time and research will prove whether or not vitamin E therapy can help improve fertility by increasing the amount of fertile mucus.

The teachers of the Ovulation Method in El Salvador, Central America, report that the people are slowly coming to realize that some form of family planning is important. For a long time, there seemed to be an innate resistance to family planning. Large families were the ideal, and, in the days when land and work were plentiful, children were considered a blessing. Men proved their virility by fathering as many children as possible—sometimes with two or more women. The women, even the unmarried ones, wanted a family as a security for their old age.

TEACHING METHODS

The teachers of the Ovulation Method in El Salvador (Figure 10–1), adapt their presentation to the people's understanding of fertility in nature. The people are told that the same God who put fertile times and infertile times in Mother Earth did the same to the human mother. And that just as success in farming depends on planting in the appropriate season, so success in family planning depends on recognizing the fertile and infertile times in the woman, appropriately. (Figure 10–1)

The comparison of Mother Nature and the woman is developed even further, as shown in Figure (10–1). First, the woman has a dry, preparatory time, and then she has a time when she feels a sensation of wetness. This sensation and the mucus flow is shown to be related to fertility, just as rain is necessary for fertile crops.

Soon the mucus and the moistness disappear, and dryness usually reappears and continues until menstruation occurs—roughly two weeks later. Note that the teachers in El Salvador place menstruation last in the explanation. They do this for many reasons, but principally, they say, because to their mind, menstruation is the last phase of the cycle, being triggered by the hormone interplay when pregnancy has not occurred in that cycle. Menstruation is described as a healthful house cleaning, one that gets rid of unused cells and tissues and leaves the uterus fresh and ready for possible occupancy in the next cycle.

Most Ovulation Centers use a chart on which colored stamps are placed to indicate the various phases of the cycle. Time has proved the value of such charts in most countries, but there are parts of the world where the local languages do not have separate words for some colors (for example, green and yellow). For this and other reasons, the teachers in Nigeria use red and blue ballpoint pens, which are in plentiful supply in the local markets. The red and blue crayons are used only to draw simple signs. Red indicates possible fertility; blue means infertility, with qualifications.

Whatever the country, cooperation between husband and wife is essential for the success of the Ovulation Method. In Nigeria the teachers stress the following:

1. The chart and the pens should always be kept in a plastic bag, and in the same place, readily accessible to both husband and wife. It is not his chart or her chart, but their chart (Figure 10–2)

Figure 10–1. In El Salvador they teach the Ovulation Method associating the fertility of the land when moist to the fertility of a woman when she is moist, resulting in a baby if the seed is planted in her body at the fertile time.

EL METODO DE LA OVULACION TAN NATURAL COMO LA MADRE TIERRA

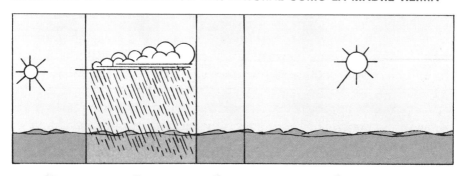

Tiempo seco infértil	Tiempo húmedo fértil	Tiempo seco encima . . . húmedo abajo . . . fértil	Tiempo seco infértil

ASI TAMBIEN LA MADRE MUJER

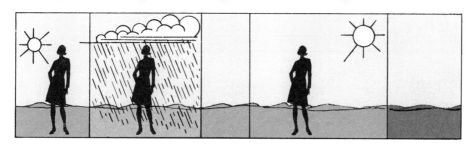

Tiempo seco infértil	Tiempo húmedo fértil	Tiempo seco encima húmedo abajo fértil		Tiempo seco infértil	REGLA
		1	2		

TIEMPO FERTIL EN LA MUJER

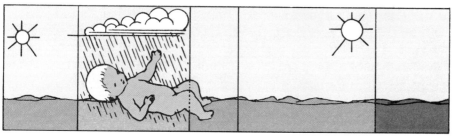

El tiempo fértil es durante el tiempo del flujo mucoso más dos días

Figure 10-1

REGLA

2. The Ovulation Method can help the love between a husband and wife grow. Reverence for each other can increase, and the baby at the breast can develop better mentally and physically because of the peace and security in the home.

An instructor in Nigeria says that she stresses that she is talking not about the fertility of the woman only, but about the combined fertility of husband and wife. The husband is encouraged to attend the initial and follow-up interviews with his wife. He is made to feel that he is involved and is not merely an onlooker.

The husband should also have a good understanding of the method. Many husbands even come to recognize when their wives are close to ovulation; they may notice either an increase in the wife's physical energy or some other less tangible change in behavior. Because the chart is kept readily accessible, the husband understands when abstinence is required. The husbands of the female instructors can also help the people by telling how they themselves feel about the Ovulation Method.

In Fiji, a special chart was designed to be used by single girls, especially high-school girls. The chart is used only to teach girls about their bodies and how they function, and the only test of effective charting is noting a girl's ability to foretell the next menstruation, which should occur approximately two weeks after she recognized her peak.

TERMINOLOGY

In Nigeria students who are unfamiliar with the word mucus are told that mucus is like the saliva that occurs in the mouth. There are two kinds of ovulation mucus. The first kind of mucus to appear after the early dry days breaks, and it is sticky and cloudy. In fact, it looks very much like the food called pap (or like cornflour). Thus for simplicity, the mucus is referred to as pap. The second kind of mucus to appear is stretchy, slippery, and clear (or almost clear). It looks like the white of a raw egg white. It feels slippery. Egg white is fertile mucus. Although pap is infertile, those who wish to avoid pregnancy are strongly advised to avoid intercourse when pap is present because pap often contains a little egg white, enough to indicate that pregnancy might occur.

The last day of the egg white and of the slippery sensation is the most important day of all. It is given a special name, the Peak. The woman cannot know that one day is the Peak until she discovers that the next day she is dry or she has a cloudy sticky mucous secretion. It is the same with the last day of the rainy season. One can only know later that it was the last day—when he sees that the following days were dry. The Peak is important because ovulation usually occurs within about 18 hours of the Peak. On the ballpoint pen chart, the Peak is designated as *Pari*, which is a local word for finish, the finish of the egg white.

The woman should use the stretch test to check the mucus. To do so, she should simply wipe herself as usual after urination. She then tries to stretch any mucus that has accumulated. She should then be easily able to decide whether the mucus is pap or egg white, or whether she is dry. The stretch test should be done every day, and after every urination. (See also pages 25–31, Figures 3–1 through 3–14).

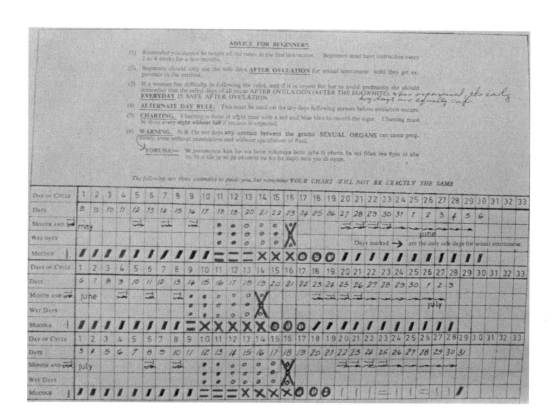

Figure 10-2. Nigeria—using symbols when charting.

The *a,b,c* mucus signs (*a*-pap, *b*-egg white, *c*-dryness) give sufficient warning of the approach of ovulation. The couple who wishes to avoid pregnancy is instructed to abstain from intercourse during the red-wet days and during the three red-zero days that follow. The abstinence must last three full days and three full nights. The couple can have intercourse safely on every dry day that follows the three red-zero days, but they must always observe the rule for egg white: Whenever egg white is seen, avoid intercourse for that day and for the three days following (see also pages 33, 34, and 80).

The *most fertile sign* gets priority over an *infertile sign:* that is, if a woman sees egg white even just once in a day and the remainder of the day is dry, she records the sign for egg white. Likewise, pap has priority over dryness, and egg white has priority over pap.

The line on the chart marked Day of Cycle should not be confused with the date of the month. (Nigeria Figure 10–2) The first day of the cycle refers to the first day of menstruation. At each new menstruation, a new line is used. In the examples on the chart (Figure 10–2), the days on which intercourse is safe are indicated by the sign.

The following terms and suggestions are used in Fiji in teaching the Ovulation Method.

- Flu-type mucus (that is, mucus that resembles the nasal discharge when one has the flu) can be described as thick, tacky, cloudy, creamy or lumpy. The number of days that that type of mucus appears may differ for each woman and in different cycles of the same woman.
- Fertile mucus can be described as like raw egg white, watery, clear, slippery, stretchy, lubricative. It can last for from one to four days, with the last day described as the Peak.

After the Peak, the woman may be dry or she may have flu type mucus again. If she is dry, she puts a green baby stamp on her chart. Whether she is wet or dry, she must wait until the fourth day after the Peak day to have intercourse. The Peak day is marked with an X whether the mucus is plentiful or scanty and whether it is noted during the whole day or during just part of the day.

DIFFICULTIES IN FAMILY PLANNING

Drunkenness is often given as an example of the problems that militate against the success of the Ovulation Method. It has been the experience of various instructors that a couple with such a problem is able to accept abstinence as a means of resolving their family planning problems, their love and respect for each other often grow, leading them to look for solutions to their basic difficulties also.

An instructor from Fiji reports that one difficulty she meets is that a number of their clients have difficulty in following the Ovulation Method for the first three

Figure 10–3. *A.* In Guatemala for rural areas they are using brown stamps for dry days, associating the dry color of the soil to the brown color of the stamps. *B.* The photograph of the mother still nursing her two-year-old son belongs to a mother who is illiterate and teaches the Ovulation Method with her husband. *C.* Her one-year record below. *D.* In Mexico—teacher with family learning method.

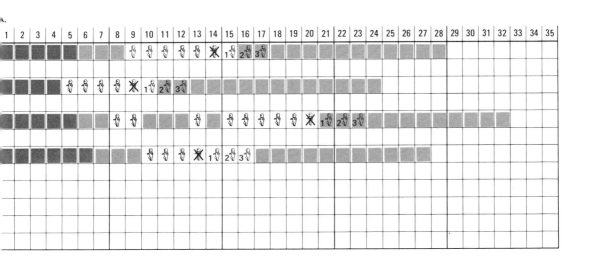

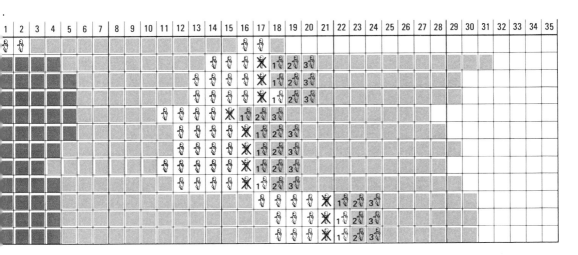

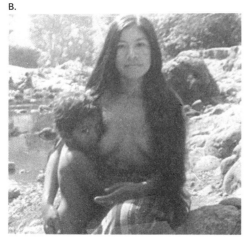

B.

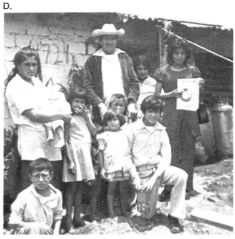

D.

months because they have been taking the Pill, which causes bodily changes that persist long after the Pill has been discontinued. (pages 94–95).

COST AND OTHER FACTORS

Another instructor in Fiji has made a cost analysis of the Ovulation Method program in her center. She estimates that the cost per person for the 1701 people they have trained was $16. For the 1059 of these people who have been registered as established (that is, using the Ovulation Method consistently and successfully), the cost worked out to $26 per person—or just about the unsubsidized cost of one year's supply of certain brands of the Pill. The established users of the Ovulation Method—and many others who are not yet registered as such—are now able to space or limit their families without further expense.

An analysis of two geographical areas in Fiji that each have a full-time instructor shows that such an arrangement is the ideal, provided that the instructor is suitably qualified and that she has suitable transportation. Both provisions are equally important. An instructor who must depend on public transportation to get to widely scattered areas may spend a whole day trying, and failing, to meet just one learner. A car enables an instructor to visit learners in various villages.

OTHER USEFUL TEACHING TOOLS AND APPROACHES

Audiovisual aids can be used to make any subject more easily understood: "I hear—I forget; I see—I remember; I do—I understand." (From script by Milross)

Audiovisual aids help:

• To stimulate discussion. After a shared experience, when the instructor and the students watch a movie together, there is greater communication.
• To stimulate and sustain interest so that the time available is used well.
• To clarify points of possible confusion.
• To deepen understanding by the visual presentation of an idea.
• To teach by example.

It should be remembered, however, that visual aids are only aids and they should not replace more personal forms of teaching.

The rest of this chapter gives outlines of the presentation of the Ovulation Method as it is made in a center in Guatemala and in a center in Fiji. Learning about some of the techniques and terms used in these centers may help instructors in other parts of the world, particularly developing countries, work more effectively with their own groups.

Guatemala

In the second class in the Guatemalan center (the first class was described on page

Figure 10-4. *A.* In India teaching female and male fertility. *B.* For achieving pregnancy. *C.* For postponing pregnancy. *D.* For choosing the sex of the baby.

Figure 10–4   **India**

A.

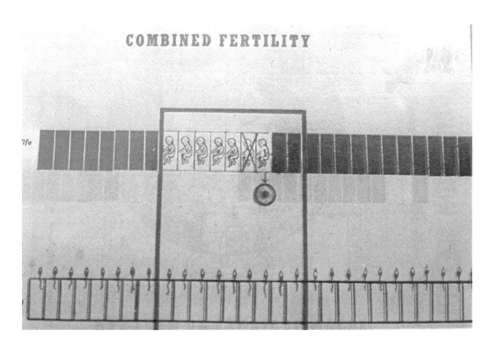

B.

Figure 10–4 (continued)

India

C.

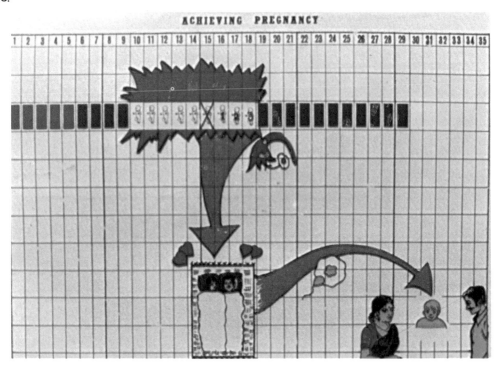

D.

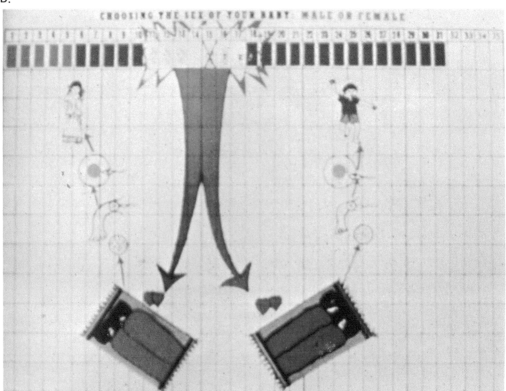

111), drawings of the female sex organs are discussed. The class ends with another discussion of the sacredness of sex and the difficulty some people have, nevertheless, in talking about sex.

In the third class, again using the dibujos (drawings), the instructor explains menstruation and discusses the male sex organs.

In the fourth class, a film strip on the Ovulation Method is shown. The film compares a woman to a bird making a nest. Cutouts of different colors of felt material are used to explain the menstrual cycle, a handy teaching tool for rural areas without electricity.

In the fourth class, photographs of the different types of mucous secretions are presented, and the women are taught to chart. The men and women are then separated into different classes. It has been found that women speak more freely about intimate matters if their husbands are not present. In the women's class, a female instructor explains charting (Figure 10-3B). A male instructor explains charting in the men's class, also emphasizing the need for the husband to respect his wife.

In the sixth, and final class, charting procedures are reviewed and the Walt Disney movie "The Human Body" is presented. The movie which is presented first in Spanish and then in Quiché (a native dialect) gives people who are unfamiliar with their bodies concrete information about anatomy and physiology. It is an excellent exposition of sex and of reproduction. It shows that each organ has its function and role. The class ends with another discussion of the sacredness of sex and the difficulty some people have, nevertheless, in talking about sex.

Fiji

In a center in Fiji, the following presentation is used.

1. Using a visual aid chart the teacher discusses the female reproductive organs using analogy. The woman prepares a "baby bag" every month—a bed, food, and a warm house. *For the bed:* The uterus becomes soft and spongy as the lining thickens. *For the food;* at ovulation, the amount of sugar in a woman's blood increases. *For the heat;* The woman's basal body temperature rises a few degrees at ovulation.

The fertility of the woman is the next topic. Mucus comes from tiny glands in the neck of the uterus, the cervix. It acts as a lubricant, to help in the transport of the sperm toward the ovum, and it nourishes the sperm. Once a sperm enters a woman's body, it takes several hours for it to complete its journey towards the ovum. A sperm is not capable of fertilizing the egg until the sperm achieves capacitation (page 32).

An egg is released monthly (during ovulation), and menstruation occurs approximately two weeks later, no matter how long the cycle is.

The man is fertile all the time—and at every phase of the woman's cycle. The man can produce sperm indefinitely. Some men are fertile into old age (see Figure 10-4A).

If pregnancy does not occur: Menstruation occurs, approximately two weeks after ovulation. The baby's bed is no longer needed, and it is shed during menstruation. The body temperature falls, and the baby's house is cooled down again. The increased sugar in the woman's blood, no longer needed, is discarded through the kidneys.

Figure 10–5

A.

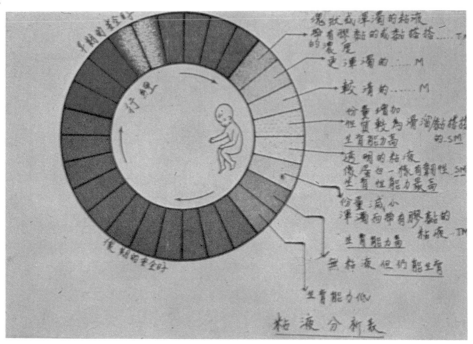

B.

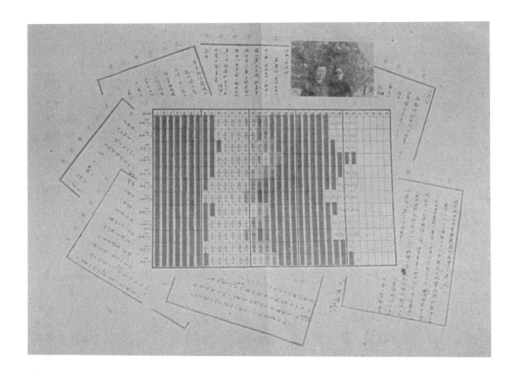

If pregnancy occurs: Menstruation does not occur because the baby is in its soft, spongy bed. The body temperature remains elevated throughout pregnancy. Sugar is present throughout pregnancy because the baby needs to be fed.

At childbirth: The bed is shed, the woman's body temperature falls, and the food is now the mother's milk, which takes the place of the sugar.

India

The enlightened guidance of Sr. Dr. Catherine Bernard and her efforts in the Tamil Nadu area are greatly appreciated by her people. Archbishop V. S. Selvanather tells us that because of its popularity, her book "Ovulation Method Training Programme" is continuously running out of stock. The ingenuity of her teaching charts is shown in Figures 10–4 A, B, C and D.

Teaching charts used in Formosa are shown in Figures 10–5 A and B.

REFERENCES

Adrian, C., Personal Communication.
Bernard, C., "Manual for Teachers of the Ovulation Method." India: Mission Press: Pondicherry.
Byrne, D., Personal Communication.
Gibbons, W., "Como Planificar Su Familia."
Jaramillo, S., Personal Communication
Levasseaur, L., Personal Communication.
McHugh, M., Personal Communication
McShane, S., Personal Communication.
McSweeney, P. L., *Birth Control O.M.* Ibadan, Nigeria: Claverianum Press.
Pitman, M., Personal Communication.
St. Marie, D., "Como Planificar Su Familia."

Figure 10–5. *A.* Circular diagram. *B.* This is a stamp chart record in Chinese with conventional colors.

11

A Statistical Evaluation
of Contraceptive Techniques

A wide variety of fertility controlling contraceptive methods, procedures and devices are today available. Although some of these methods have been in use for hundreds of years (Fallopius is said by Bernstein [1974] to have described the penile sheath in 1564) much research has been done since the early 1960's on the development of hormone-based contraceptives (OC) and intrauterine devices (IUD). Though traditional methods are still being employed, both contraceptive users and personnel of family planning agencies appear to have switched, in significant proportions, to newer methods. Table 1 presents information on contraceptive choice from the National Fertility Studies of 1955 and 1965 as well as the selections of over 27,000 new patients of Los Angeles County family planning institutions for the year 1972. The 1955 data show 75 percent of users selected condom, diaphragm or rhythm methods. By 1965, with the introduction of OCs, roughly 40 percent selected condom, diaphragm or rhythm with 27 percent on OCs. By 1972 over 85 percent of users chose OC or IUD while less than 5 percent of users employed condom, diaphragm or rhythm. The older methods are still occasionally being used but OC and IUD are today's predominant selections.

TABLE 11–1. Selected Contraceptive Methods (%).

METHOD	1955	1965	1970	1972
OC	0	27	34	64
IUD	0	0	7	23
Condom	27	18	14	1
Diaphragm	25	10	6	3
Rhythm	22	13	1	1

GOALS

All fertility controlling procedures, from surgical sterilization to abstinence have as their goal the prevention or delay of pregnancy. With this motivation much research has been done in the last 20 years to determine the safety and effectiveness of various contraceptive procedures and devices. In addition to their primary contraceptive effects most of these procedures have side effects, effects on the human body, behavior or emotions beyond that of preventing or delaying pregnancy. These effects vary in severity from the difficulty (or impossibility) of reversing surgical sterilization, to the sometimes psychologically disruptive effects that accompany last-minute insertion of foam or diaphragm. One aspect of the evaluation of contraceptive techniques is to determine and evaluate these side effects. The severity of side effects is often reflected in the proportion of users that persist, or fail to persist, in their use of a particular technique over a significant period of time.

EVALUATION METHODOLOGY

Persons or organizations interested in research projects designed to evaluate contraceptive techniques typically begin by defining a relevant population (almost always women)[1] for whom the method is appropriate. A group of women is selected from this population for the research project. The participants are assumed to be fertile, not pregnant and as volunteers they are willing, cooperative and motivated to varying degrees. The investigators describe their research samples in terms of age, marital status, number of children, and often in terms of education, race and socio-economic status also. Most research projects select a minimum duration of study, a fixed time-period over which all participants should be observed. It is obvious that one month is too short an interval, and it is also obvious that extended programs make increased demands on research time and finances as well as participant cooperation. Many recent projects have 2- or 3-year durations and publish results based on 12 and 24 month periods.

TERMINATIONS

In Tietze's (1971) definitive work on the evaluation of contraceptive methods he enumerates the reasons, beyond accidental pregnancy, for termination of participants from these researches. Some of these reasons apply almost equally well to most contraceptive methods, for example, "Planning of Pregnancy"[2] and "Loss to follow-up", the woman who fails to meet her clinic appointments and whom researchers are unable to contact by mail or phone. In almost all studies some women are also terminated for "Personal Reasons".

Other participants are terminated for reasons related to the specific method being evaluated, such as "Expulsion of IUD." Some researchers classify the various categories of termination as "Use-related" and "Nonrelated" while others describe "User Failures," "Method Failures," "Biological Failures" and "Personal Failures."

DATA COLLECTED

Participants in studies evaluating contraceptive procedures are observed periodically by investigators and classified as either continuing in the study or terminated. The

---

[1] With the recent exception of vasectomy, Bernstein's (1976) statement about the condom still holds, " . . . This 400-year-old device is still the only male contraceptive available . . . "

[2] In most studies the percent users terminated for 'Planning Pregnancy' is far below that of 'Accidental Pregnancy'.

terminations are broken down by accidental pregnancies and other reasons. This information should be collected monthly, but the results are often presented in 6-month intervals, 6, 12, 18, 24 months and longer. In the analysis and presentation of results terminations are classified by reason or groups of reasons and by duration on the method. Duration on the method is presented in various ways, from women/months of use, monthly termination rates and more commonly, the cumulative termination rate, that is, the percent of accidental pregnancies per year. Continuation rates, the proportion or percentage of women still employing the method is often presented, and occasionally Pearl's (Jay) formula, the number of pregnancies per 100 women years (an older statistic), is encountered.

INTERPRETATION OF RESULTS

In his "Statistical Evaluations of Contraceptive Methods" (1971) Tietze describes several levels for evaluating contraceptive methods.

1. "Theoretical effectiveness or its capacity to reduce the risk of accidental pregnancy under laboratory conditions, taking into account anatomic and physiologic responses but not psychologic factors.
2. "Use-effectiveness or its performance under real life conditions. Including any accidental pregnancies during regular or irregular use of the method under study but excluding pregnancies following discontinuation of contraception or adoption of another method.
3. "Extended use-effectiveness, including all accidental pregnancies occurring after discontinuation of the method under study while the woman is still at risk."

Theoretical effectiveness as such is difficult or impossible to assess directly and may be thought of as the biological and physiological effectiveness of the method in the absence of all human error. Theoretical effectiveness is estimated from the evaluation of results of groups of human users under ordinary error-filled-home-life conditions and it is seen as an upper limit of use-effectiveness. Use-effectiveness is the practical evaluation of the technique assessed in the presence of human error contributed in varying and unknown amounts by the women, their partners and possibly the researchers as well.

TYPICAL RESULTS FOR DIFFERENT METHODS

In 1974 Ogra et al. published their analysis of OC use-effectiveness for a group of 2000 women over the period 1962–1968. Their group was described as having a mean age of 24.9 years and a mean parity of 2.5 children. The group was also described as 54.2 percent lower class, 36.3 percent low-middle, and 9.5 percent as middleclass. The accidental pregnancy rates are presented as cumulative termination rates for 1, 2 and 3 years in Table 2. Highest rates of accidental pregnancy were found among the youngest group of women (less than 20 years). These accidental pregnancy rates were almost all *below 5 percent over the three-year period*, and decreased consistently with increased age of user.

TABLE 11–2 Cumulative Termination and Continuation Rates.

AGE	ACCIDENTAL PREGNANCIES (%) CUMULATIVE TERMINATION RATE			CUMULATIVE CONTINUATION RATE (%)	
	1	2	3	1	3 (YEARS)
15–19	2.3	4.2	5.3	75.6	38.3
20–24	1.4	2.0	2.3	81.8	48.9
25–29	1.3	1.3	1.8	83.7	61.9
30–34	0.8	0.8	0.8	88.0	68.5
35 +	0.0	0.0	—*	75.6	—*

* Samples too small to follow further

Women 35 and over had no accidental pregnancies. Ogra's analysis did not reveal any systematic relationship between number of previous children and accidental pregnancy. The last two columns of Table 2 present the cumulative continuation rates, that is the proportion of women continuing the use of OCs after 1 and 3 years of use. The 12-month continuation rates ranged from about 75 percent to 90 percent, while the 3-year continuation rates vary from a low of less than 40 percent for the under-20 group to a high 88 percent continuation rate for the 30 to 34 group. In conclusion this study suggests that OCs had a very high use-effectiveness rate and that older women tend to persist in their use of OCs to a much greater extent than women under 25 years of age.

TABLE 11–3. 12-Month Cumulative Rates (%).

AGE	PREGNANCIES		ALL TERMINATIONS	
	IUD	OC	IUD	OC
Under 20	9.1	15.1	27.4	50.0
20–24	6.7	4.6	29.5	30.9
25–29	3.6	8.3	19.6	31.6
30+	0.5	6.4	9.9	44.6

Tietze and Lewit published a comparison of the use-effectiveness of the IUD and OC in 1971. About 2,900 women in three localities, Atlanta, Brooklyn and Buffalo were included in the study, approximately 1,200 starting with the IUD and the remaining 1,700 on OCs.

Table 11–3 presents 12-month cumulative termination rates for accidental pregnancies with IUD and OC and also the gross termination rates, that is, all women terminated for any reason from their initial contraceptive selection for the 12-month period. In comparing the OC results with those of Ogra it appears immediately that the 12-month accidental pregnancy rates are considerably higher than the previous study. In fact the 12-month pregnancy rates of this study are higher than the 36-month pregnancy rates of the previous work. As in Ogra's study Tietze also found the highest accidental pregnancy rates with his youngest group of users, and this finding was consistent with IUD users as well as the OC group. In general the IUD group seems to have significantly fewer accidental pregnancies than the group employing OC. Tietze and Lewit concluded that women selecting the IUD as a contraceptive method were older and more persistent in their use of contraceptives than those selecting OCs.

In 1974 Jain presented an analysis of results of about 16,000 U.S. users of the TCu-200 IUD. Table 11–4 presents the 12-month cumulative termination rates for their group as well as additional groups of IUD users in Finland and Korea. Overall termination rates are broken down by type for accidental pregnancies, IUD expulsion and removal of IUD as well as the percent retaining and continuing with the IUD. The accidental pregnancy rate for the three groups was quite low, from a little over 1 percent to a little less than 3 percent for the 12-month period involving approximately 20,000 users.

TABLE 11–4.   TCu-200 IUD 12-Month Cumulative Rates (%).

TYPE OF TERMINATION	U.S.	FINLAND	KOREA
Total	25.5	10.9	31.3
Pregnancy	2.6	1.6	1.1
Expulsion	7.3	2.2	6.0
Removal	15.6	7.1	24.3
Retentions	74.4	89.1	68.7
Insertions	16,345	2,689	1,050

The highest accidental pregnancy rate (2.6 percent) of the U.S. group may be related to the fact that it was the youngest group, with an approximate mean age of 25 years, while the Korean group had the lowest accidental pregnancy rate (1.1 percent) with a mean age of approximately 33 years. It should be emphasized that all accidental pregnancy rates were very low. Jain's 24-month results for the U.S. group reveal that the 20 to 25 age group had the highest accidental pregnancy rate of 5.7 percent, the 15–19 year group slightly lower at 5.3 percent while women over 30 had 2-year accidental pregnancy rates of less than 3 percent. All three groups had significant proportions (7–24 percent) of IUDs removed during the first year. These removals were the greatest single termination factor and were performed for a variety of reasons including persistent bleeding and/or pain, planning pregnancy, and other medical and personal reasons. In the first 12-month period 1.9 percent were removed due to 'Planning Pregnancy'.

Lane, Arceo and Sobrero in 1976 published a study of the use of the diaphragm and jelly contraceptive method with a group of over 2,000 users. The group was characterized as young (more than 50 percent under 25), unmarried (71 percent), never pregnant (72 percent) and 92 percent white. Table 11–5 presents the 12-month cumulative termination rates for accidental pregnancy and for termination for 'Personal Reasons'. Cumulative termination rates are presented for several age groups. The 12-month use-effectiveness rate for all ages combined was 1.9 percent accidental pregnancies. Lane et al also present data from seven other studies of the diaphragm method, each involving more than 500 users, and in these studies accidental pregnancy rates vary from a low of 2.4 percent to a high of 25 percent for a 12-month study interval. These investigators feel that if a contraceptive program is routinely administered with "cursory care" and minimal supervision, that one can expect higher accidental pregnancy rates. They feel that their own success with this method was due, at least in part, to "the level of instruction, which bolstered the patient's self-confidence, and a mechanism for continuing supervision. The participation of personnel who believed in the method and who possessed the skill and patience to teach it was crucial." These investigators also feel that the factors of quality of instruction and user motivation may account for the fact that their study did not show the higher rate of accidental pregnancy for young users that is typical of other investigations.

TABLE 11–5.   Termination Rates Diaphragm (%).

AGE	ACCIDENTAL PREGNANCIES	PERSONAL REASONS*
13–17	1.9	29.7
18–20	2.3	17.1
21–24	2.0	12.3
25–29	2.9	13.5
30–34	3.0	9.1
35+	0.0	6.0

* Personal Reasons included rejection of diaphragm as messy, difficult to insert, because of objection of partner or just selection of another method.

In Bernstein's (1974) study of the use-effectiveness of condom, diaphragm and foam he states that risk in condom use is dependent primarily on user care and motivation (which is true with most methods) and that risk due to a defective device is much less than 1 percent. Pregnancy rates from several studies are cited as varying from 4–36/100 women years of exposure. Tietze estimates that the theoretical effectiveness of the condom is probably equivalent to that of the IUD and he also emphasizes the role of user motivation. Bernstein also describes a study of about 3000 users of vaginal foam that resulted in an accidental pregnancy rate of 4.3/100 women years of exposure.

In 1970 Tietze published "Ranking of Contraceptive Methods by Levels of Effectiveness". All widely used contraceptive methods were evaluated by theoretical effectiveness estimated from numerous studies. The methods were divided into four groups: Most Effective, Highly Effective, Less Effective and Least Effective Techniques. Methods classified as Most Effective included tubal sterilization, vasectomy, combined and sequential OCs and the Temperature Rhythm method. This TR method involves the determination of ovulation by measuring and recording of basal body temperature and requires restriction of coitus to the postovulatory phase of the cycle. Coitus must be avoided not only prior to ovulation but also in the postovulatory phase if the temperature indication of ovulation is in doubt. Tietze mentions one study under these conditions that reported a single method failure in 17,500 cycles. It is interesting to note that he also reports 34 pregnancies occurring in a group of about 20,000 sterilized women and 15 pregnancies involving 3,330 vasectomized males.

Classified as Highly Effective Methods are the diaphragm, IUD and condom, all of which Tietze estimates to have a theoretical effectiveness of 1 percent to 3 percent method failures per year.

Chemical contraceptives, foams, jellies, creams, tablets and suppositories, calendar rhythm and coitus interruptus are classified as Less Effective. Of coitus interruptus Tietze says, "its effectiveness should not be discounted since it was the method mainly responsible for the early historical decline in birth rates among the peoples of northern and western Europe." The Least Effective category includes the douche and continued breast-feeding. Table 11–5 presents the methods and theoretical effectiveness estimates for the two highest categories.

TABLE 11–6. Ranking of Contraceptive Methods.

METHOD	THEORETICAL EFFECTIVENESS
MOST EFFECTIVE	
Tubal Sterilization	0.08
Vasectomy	0.15
OC (combined type)	0.07
OC (sequential type)	0.34
Temperature Rhythm	1.2
HIGHLY EFFECTIVE	
IUD	1.5–3.0
Diaphragm	1.5–3.0
Condom	1.5–3.0
OC (continuous) "minipill"	2.3

A study by Ryder (1973) approaches the topic of contraceptive use-effectiveness from the viewpoint of user satisfaction, or dissatisfaction, which is an approach quite different from other works discussed here. Ryder worked with data collected in the 1970 National Fertility Study, interviews conducted with a national sample of 6,752 ever-married women. Respondents were queried as to their contraceptive behaviors, whether or not contraceptives were used, what method or methods and whether the intent of contraception was to *delay* or *prevent* pregnancy. Respondents were also asked whether or not they had been successful in their contraceptive intentions over the previous 12-month period. Data were analyzed with respect to type of contraceptive method, intent, age, race, religion and other variables. Figure 11–1 presents the overall method-specific failure rates by intent.

These results indicate that women who intend to *prevent* pregnancy are more successful than those who wish to *delay* and that the more modern contraceptive methods (OC and IUD) are considerably more effective than all others, while douche, foam and rhythm are less effective. Ryder notes that his failure rates are greater than would be expected from an evaluation of the theoretical effectivenesses of the methods and describes one of the reasons, "Suppose, for example, a woman began use of the pill, but abandoned it because of side effects. Should she fail to begin using another method promptly, the likelihood is that she would become pregnant. That pregnancy would be recorded in our procedure as a pill failure." This is an example of Tietze's "Extended Use-effectiveness." Ryder goes on to emphasize a conclusion of other contraceptive investigators: "It seems to us most important to recognize the extent to which the outcome of use is the *joint consequence* of method characteristics and user characteristics."

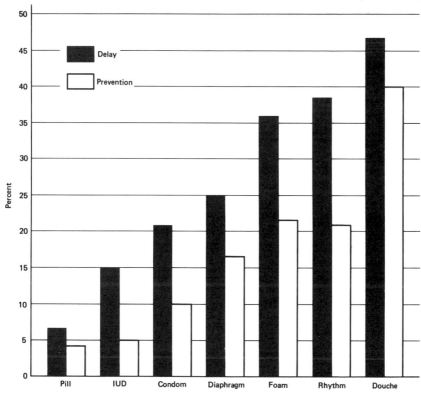

Figure 11-1. Contraceptive failures in first 12 months of use, by method and intent of contraception.

Variables found to be related to failure rates in this study included:

1. *Intent.* Women using contraceptives with the intent to delay rather than prevent pregnancy have significantly higher failure rates.

2. *Age.* Younger women have considerably higher failure rates.

3. *Past history of contraceptive failure.* Past history of contraceptive failure is associated with increased probability of future failure.

In comparing this study with National Fertility Studies over a period of 15 years Ryder concluded that the contraceptive failure rate *has been reduced by at least 50 percent* over this period, and he attributes this increase in contraceptive success almost entirely to the large increase in women using OCs.

This large increase in contraceptive effectiveness has not been without price, however. As the number of OC users increases, and as the proportion of long-term OC users increases we find more and more studies devoted to the side effects of these pervasive and persistent disturbances of the endocrine system. In a survey by Hume (1978) these side effects varied from increased mortality rates among OC users, especially but not exclusively related to thromboembolisms and myocardial infarctions, increased liver tumors, increased incidence of hypertension, elevated blood pressure, increased incidence of venereal disease, loss of interest in sex, impairment of normal coping mechanisms and infertility after discontinuance of OCs. Concern over the long-term side effects of OCs is such that it has given rise to an editorial in the prestigious British medical publication *Lancet,* "Mortality Associated with the Pill." As the number of long-term users increases it seems likely that more disturbing findings will emerge.

In one of earliest evaluations of the Ovulation Method (OM), Weisman, Foliaki, Billings, and Billings (1972) describe the instruction and application of the OM with a group on the Pacific island community of Tonga. Of 395 women instructed in the OM 331 couples elected to continue in its use. As the OM is always described as a method of fertility control which may enhance the probability of pregnancy as well as lower it, a number of women (18) included were attempting to achieve pregnancy. As with other methods the investigators recorded numerous instances of irregular use of OM or 'deliberate carelessness' of the users. Accidental pregnancies were classified as biological or method failure if the couple was felt to understand and use the method properly, or as user or personal failure if it was felt that pregnancy resulted from incorrect understanding of the method on the part of the couple. For the 50 cases where the woman was impulsive, or she and her partner had intercourse during her fertile period, the pregnancies were classed as "ignored indication of possible fertility." The group of 282 women using OM for a total of 2,503 months recorded two cases of user failure and one case of method failure.

In 1976 Ball reported a study of the OM with 124 women of rural Victoria, Australia. The women were from 20 to 39 years of age with about 75 percent of the group 30 or over. Ball reports a total of 21 accidental pregnancies, with 4 pregnancies due to biological or method failure. The Pearl rate for method failure was 2.9/100 women years while the Pearl rate for the total 21 accidental pregnancies was 15.5/100 women years.

At the 1978 Australian *International Conference on the Ovulation Method* a number of preliminary reports of ongoing applications of the OM were presented. From Korea, Stewart reported that over 8,000 females on OM had produced a 3 percent unexplained failure rate. Kearns of El Salvador reported that 20 percent of her 700 couples using OM became pregnant as the result of "taking a chance" but report only one method failure. Bernard, studying 3,000 users of OM in India reported seven user failures and no method failures. These reports are fragmentary and incomplete, but when these studies are completed and their results analyzed they should provide a great deal of much needed additional information on the use-effectiveness of the OM.

In a recent publication of a pilot study of OM use-effectiveness Klaus (1977) followed closely the procedures outlined by Tietze and Lewit (1971) in terms of data collection and presentation. Of 630 women instructed in the OM 135 agreed to be users. This group had a mean age of approximately 30 years and were primarily urban dwellers of high school or higher education levels. When accidental pregnancy occurred users were queried as to whether or not they followed the method conscientiously, and depending on their responses they were classified as Biological Failure or Personal Failure.

Table 11–7 presents Klaus' 12 and 24-month accidental pregnancy rate for biological, personal and total failures. Biological (method) failure rates for 12 and 24-months are .072 percent and .517 percent. Personal failure rates were 1.23 percent and 1.38 percent for 12 and 24 months. The standard procedure for most investigators is to combine biological and personal failures for a total accidental pregnancy rate. Lane (1976) reported that 22 of her 37 accidental pregnancies used the diaphragm, "inconsistently or not at all." Klaus followed the combinatorial approach and her total accidental pregnancy rate for 12 months was 1.30 percent, for 24 months 1.896 percent. All of these rates are quite low, on the order of the lowest 12 and 24 accidental pregnancy rates reported for other methods. Klaus' work suggests that the OM might be included in Tietze's Most Effective category, however the small number of participants in this study most strongly suggests the need of continued additional research in the evaluation of the OM.

TABLE 11-7.   Termination Rates OM.

TERMINATION FOR	CUMULATIVE RATE (%)	
	12 MO.	24 MO.
Biological Failure	0.072	0.517
Personal Failure	1.231	1.379
Total	1.303	1.896

In order to assess whether women of different countries and cultural backgrounds are capable of detecting the signs and symptoms associated with ovulation, in 1975 the World Health Organization initiated a multi-centred clinical evaluation of the Ovulation Method in India, the Philippines, New Zealand, Ireland and El Salvador. The second purpose of the clinical evaluation was to determine the use-effectiveness and the theoretical effectivensss of the Ovulation Method in women who are capable of detecting changes in the cervical mucus. At the end of 1978 the preliminary results of this study indicated that from the first month of instruction 93% of the subjects confirmed their ability to recognize their mucus pattern of fertility. Eight hundred (870) women contributed 2,685 cycles of exposure and 40 pregnancies occurred, i.e., 19.4 pregnancies per 100 woman years. However, only three of the pregnancies occurred when the method appeared to be used correctly. Thus, the theoretical effectiveness of the Ovulation Method is 98.5% effective in this study. These figures agree with the findings of other studies of the Ovulation Method. For further information see Appendix (1).

In summary, it is clear from the evidence that today's women, and today's families, have access to a variety of highly effective contraceptive methods. It is also obvious that most, if not all, of these methods are accompanied by one or more side effects with varying degrees of physiological and/or psychological discomfort or hazard. The side effects may range from death due to thrombo-embolism caused by oral contraceptives, the perforated uterus which occasionally accompanies insertion of an IUD, through increased bleeding and physical pain, to the psychological discomfort which may accompany periodically being required to refrain from certain types of sexual activity. These are the facts upon which the women and families of today must base their personal contraceptive decisions.

REFERENCES

Ball, M. 1976 Rural Victoria, reported by Hume, K. "The Ovulation Method of Natural Family Planning." *Journal of the Irish Medical Association,* 1977, **70,** 208–214

Bernard, C. Preliminary results presented at the International Conference on the Ovulation Method, Melbourne, Australia, 1978.

Bernstein, G. S. "Conventional Methods of Contraception: Condom, Diaphragm, and Vaginal foam." *Clinical Obstetrics and Gynecology,* 1974, **17**, 21–33.

Dolack, Sr. Leona, OSF, RN "Study Confirms Values of Ovulation Method," *Hospital Progress,* August, 1978, 64–66.

Hume, K. "Physical Consequences of Contraception: The Metabolic Mischief of the Pill." Paper delievered at the International Conference, Humanae Vitae, Melbourne, Australia, 1978.

Jain, A. K. "Safety and Effectiveness of Intrauterine Devices."*Contraception,* 1975, **11**, 242–259.

Kearns, F. Preliminary results presented at the International Conference on the Ovulation Method, Melbourne, Australia, (El Salvador), 1978.

Klaus, H., Goebel, J., Woods, R., Castles, M. and Zimny, G. "Use-effectiveness and Analysis of Satisfaction Levels with the Billings Ovulation Method. Two Year Pilot Study." *Fertility and Sterility Journal,* **28**, No. 10, October 1977.

Lane, M. E., Arceo, R. and Sobrero, A. "Successful Use of the Diaphragm and Jelly by a Young Population: Report of a Clinical Study." *Family Planning Perspectives,* 1976, **8**, 81–86.

Ogra, S., Feldman, J. and Lippes, J. Use-effectiveness of Oral Contraceptives by Demographic Characteristics." *Fertility and Sterility,* 1971, **21**, 677–682.

Ryder, N. "Contraceptive Failure in the United States." *Family Planning Perspectives,* 1973, **5**, 133–142.

Stewart, T. Preliminary Results Presented at the International Conference on the Ovulation Method, Melbourne, Australia, (Happy Family Movement–Korea), 1978.

Tietze, C. "Ranking of Contraceptive Methods by levels of Effectiveness," *Advances in Planned Parenthood,* 1971, **6**, 117–123.

Tietze, C. and Lewit, S. "Use-effectiveness of Oral and Intrauterine Contraception." *Fertility and Sterility,* 1971, **22**, 508–513.

Tietze, C. and Lewit, S. "Statistical Evaluation of Contraceptive Methods." *Clinical Obstetrics and Gynecology,* 1974, **17**, 121–138.

Weismann, M., Foliaki, L., Billings, E. and Billings, J. A Trial of the Ovulation Method of Family Planning in Tonga. *The Lancet,* 1972, **14**, 813–816.

World Health Organization Seventh Annual Report, November 1978 (unpublished document).

12

Psychological Aspects of Birth Control: Woman's Freedom to Choose

Attempts to limit conception or to control and space births have a major role in human sexuality. The search for practical methods of family planning began centuries ago and is documented elsewhere in much detail (Williams, 1977; Seaman and Seaman, 1977). Many methods proposed and used even in recent times have brought painful scarring, and humiliating experiences to the woman forced to tamper with the natural order of heterosexual relations. It is ironic to realize, amid so much endeavor to control a natural function of the woman's body—pregnancy—that women have played such a passive role.

In 1956, synthetic progesterone and estrogen compounds were tested as contraceptives for Puerto Rican and Haitian women. The short-term results were encouraging and chemical regulation of the reproductive cycle was soon a billion dollar business. Chapter 8 explains in detail the action of these contraceptive pills and some of the effects of upsetting the delicate balance of the endocrine system with the brain. As always, any adverse consequences of birth control methods have been borne by women. The latest "benefits" of science, the Pill and the IUD, are producing an increasing number of pathological conditions and debilitating psychological effects. The long-term effects of most modern forms of birth control are yet unknown, yet the need for effective birth control is obvious. More and more women are engaged in dual roles. Women's contribution to society has changed from one of being an instrument of procreation toward one of being an active productive member of the society. Social structures are changing such that women are entering the legal, political, and economic systems in ways not seen before. One of the most important factors contributing to this new freedom is the control of fertility. Not only have the means become more available but women are now taking a more active voice in the use of such methods. "Unforturnately, women all over are walking out of clinics and doctors' offices with methods of birth control that they have not really thought about or clearly chosen, and are not sure how to use." (Boston Women's Health Book Collective, 1976, page 182). It is estimated that 12 to 15 million women around the world take the Pill. There is a tremendous need for women to participate more actively in the selection and control of any of the birth control methods they use.

The methods of birth control currently available, and the various side effects associated with each were discussed in Chapter 8. The method a woman chooses is a function of its effectiveness in meeting her needs both physiologically and psychologically. The psychological effects on the user of any method of birth control are a function of (1) effectiveness; (2) convenience and esthetics of use; (3) effect of use on the woman's health; and (4) religious, ethical, moral and cultural concerns of both partners in the relationship. The order of importance of these factors obviously will differ from couple to couple. Mechanical methods such as the IUD are now being viewed with skepticism because of physical dangers and the covert psychological effect due to its probable abortifacient action. Other barrier methods (diaphragm, condom, spermicides) are felt by some to be unesthetic, inhibiting the spontaneity of sexual intercourse, somewhat cumbersome and not totally eradicating the fear of pregnancy. Sterilization, whether for medical reason or personal choice, involves physical and psychological changes both in men and women that are not fully understood. Physical reactions to oral contraceptives are unquestionably related to the higher and constant levels of estrogen and progesterone than are normally produced by the body. Consequently, a panic reaction has set in against use of oral contraceptives. Contributing to this reaction is the widespread discussion of contraceptives and contraception in newspapers, magazines, on radio and TV and in conversation. It is not surprising, that user reaction is influenced by the popular media treatment of fact and rumor. In the OM centers women state that their husbands did not want them on the Pill because of reports of its published ill effects. This concern is very flattering for the wife whose husband does not want her to risk her health, especially when he is willing to accept a period of abstinence in the middle of the cycle for the sake of her physical and emotional well being.

The number of side effects associated with available means of birth control have led to a heightened interest in more natural means of birth control -"... one that involved no chemicals, nothing worn inside our vagina or uterus, had no side effects, was shared equally, and was perfectly effective" (Boston Women's Health Book Collective, 1976, page 207). These methods depend upon the woman's recognition of her own bodily signs. All are based on recognition that there are fertile periods and nonfertile periods in the cycle. Although the physiological side effects of natural methods are negligible there is still a measurable risk of pregnancy. Women electing to use the Ovulation Method or other natural methods involving periodic abstinence should be provided with information about the effectiveness of the method in preventing pregnancy compared to chemical and barrier methods as provided in Chapter 11. In that way they may choose on a rational basis which method is preferable, which risks they are willing to take with their bodies, or which benefits are most important. Natural family planning is being taught in formal courses literally world wide, in junior high schools, high schools and colleges, in seminars and informal groups. Some teaching is under Church sponsorship and some is not. In adult teaching situations the interaction of family planning and marriage is, of course, of profound importance. In following a natural method both man and woman learn that the woman is only fertile for about 100 hours every month. It is not surprising that a woman resents having to take powerful medication daily or having to wear a mechanical device for years when she needs to prevent pregnancy only during a few days in every cycle. The knowledge that the man is always fertile and the woman only occasionally fertile serves to take the burden of the responsibility off the woman and have it shared by the two of them. This mutual responsibility serves to remove the burden that has been on the woman for many generations.

The Ovulation Method is a challenge. Not only does a couple have to learn how their bodies function, they also have to study the pattern of mucous secretions and practice restraint during fertile periods. This requires some sacrifice. However, most people are willing and able to meet this challenge.

Users and advocates of natural family planning come from a diversity of cultures, nations and races. Religious, ethical and moral concerns, of course, are important factors in any expressed reaction to birth control. It is a matter of record that the natural methods of family planning were early endorsed as being not contrary to Catholic doctrine, and in consequence the teaching of natural methods has the possibility for Church sponsorship. The Ovulation Method in particular is a development of the Doctors Billings, themselves Catholic. The first widespread teaching was done by Catholic missionaries. Currently, the method is beginning to reach many arenas. A recent report (McKay, 1978) indicated the success by a Planned Parenthood Clinic in teaching the Ovulation Method. In contrast to most data provided on the Ovulation Method, where the population is primarily Catholic with an average family size of four, the Planned Parenthood population included over 50 percent single and independent women with 75 percent childless by choice. The appeal of a natural effective method is thus being evidenced in a wide diversity of women.

Much is being written today about the reactions of women using the Ovulation Method, or other natural methods, as a means of fertility control (Jackson; Christenson 1977). The reports are unanimous in attesting to the psychological attractiveness and intellectual satisfaction experienced by women in developed as well as developing countries. It is very interesting, in fact, to note reports which seem so similar both from developing and developed countries. A missionary told about a very poor and humble couple who learned the method and who during the fertile phase said that they treat each other like they used to when they were engaged. In the developed countries, couples also admit that abstinence is not necessarily easy but then when they were engaged, it wasn't easy either.

An often reported outcome of use of the Ovulation Method is a more meaningful relationship and the improvement of communication between husband and wife. The sharing of the intimate knowledge of the woman's menstrual cycle opens the door for better communication in other areas. Many couples are now sending their older children to learn natural family planning not only for biological and physiological education, but because they can foresee the advantages of this knowledge when their children contemplate marriage. Future generations will be able to plan their families in a natural way without the risks their parents experienced. It also gives them an opportunity to learn before marriage about their cyclic fertility without the additional pressure of adapting to a new married life.

An observer in Central America related that just as the artificial methods have secondary harmful effects, the natural methods have secondary beneficial effects, so much so, that child spacing becomes a secondary effect. The primary effect that he has seen is how it unites the couple. A man and a woman have sexual relations for many reasons, two of which are mutual love and to procreate children. When a couple has the number of children that they feel they can afford, sexual relations, particularly from the woman's point of view, often become a worrying and fearful experience that she no longer enjoys due to the fear of pregnancy. When her husband becomes affectionate, she reacts angrily or is tired, and as a consequence, not much pleasure emanates for him or for her. However, once the couple understand their fertility, they not only have relations more often but with greater pleasure, which is obviously conducive to better marital life. The children in turn benefit greatly from this harmony in the home. Most of the people who use this method in the mission in Central America are not married, but after introducing them to the Ovulation Method and making them aware of their power of fertililty, they come to the missionary saying, "We are getting along fine now, there just isn't any reason not to get married." Another surprising development resulting from this fertility knowledge is that not only does the woman no longer refuse sexual relations during the infertile phase, but for that culture, the unheard of occurs, she becomes more affectionate, the initiator of sexual relations.

Occurrence of Pregnancy with Ovulation Method

As described in detail in Chapter 11, a wide variety of contraceptive methods, procedures and devices are today available. The success or failure of each of these methods is closely associated not only with the reliability of the method, but to a great degree also with the reliability of the user. That is, no matter how reliable a method is, it cannot succeed unless certain rules are followed rigidly for each of them. For this reason, it is important to make a distinction between method failure and user failure. The reasons for method failure have been discussed in Chapter 11. In view of user failure with OM, Dr. Billings recommends that the teaching staff discuss possible pregnancy with each couple from the very beginning, so that they may contemplate how they would handle an unexpected pregnancy resulting from disregard of the OM rules. In many cases involving married couples, there is no serious resentment when an unplanned pregnancy occurs. One reason for this may be that the couple knew they were taking a chance by having sexual relations during a fertile period. "Next time we'll be more careful", or "we knew we were taking a chance", are their usual comments. It is amazing how many couples return to the Ovulation Method after the birth of their "unplanned baby". Very often the cause of pregnancy is that either the husband or the wife really want another child, but do not openly admit that desire. Other couples become careless in their record keeping, feeling that they have mastered the method and no longer need to keep such careful daily records. Sometimes a marital problem exists, and the lack of communication and cooperation results in a pregnancy.

From the women encountered in OM centers, as well as from stories related worldwide, results strongly indicate that the Ovulation Method has brought considerable satisfaction to the users, namely safety, simplicity, esthetic satisfaction, and compatibility with religious, moral and ethical concepts on which their value systems are built. Probably the most compelling rationale for the increasing use of the Ovulation Method is that it relies on the expanding scientific knowledge about human reproduction, in contrast to the expedient use of chemical contraceptives and IUDs, which has already hindered, far too long, the exploration of safer alternative methods.

REFERENCES

Boston Women's Health Book Collective, *Our Bodies, Ourselves.* New York; Simon and Schuster, 1976.

Christenson, Nordis, *The Christian Couple.* Minnesota; Bethany Fellowship, 1977.

Jackson, Leah, Personal Communication.

McKay, Marsha, "The Ovulation Method and Planned Parenthood," *Planned Parenthood News,* Vol. 1, Issue 3, June–Sept. 1978, Program in Focus, **4,** 1978.

St. Marie, Dennis. Personal communication.

Seaman, B. and Seaman, G. *Women and the Crisis in Sex Hormones.* New York; Rawson Associates Publishers, 1977.

Williams, J. H. *Psychology of Women: Behavior in a Biosocial Context.* New York; W. W. Norton and Company, 1977.

Afterword

For the past five years it has been my privilege to know Mercedes Wilson and to have taught hundreds of couples with her. I can now say that I have learned more about the cycle of the normal woman from Mrs. Wilson than I ever learned from books.

In summing up the Wayne State meeting on Ovulation in April, 1977, a European doctor said, "It looks to me that the new methods have now become old and that the old method has now become new.

Technology will never reach every woman in the world with a pill, or a coil, or even a thermometer. But in the next ten years we will reach every woman in the world with a concept, "When you are dry the sperm will die; when you are wet a baby you can get."

Mrs. Mercedes Wilson has become the premier teacher of the Ovulation Method in the United States. She is president of World Organization Ovulation Method Billings. The University of Puerto Rico has awarded her an honorary doctor's degree. Her greatest contribution has been the introduction of colored stamps in charting the menstrual cycle. These stamps convey the same meaning in every language, in all eighty countries in which the method is now taught. "If she spotted, if she bled, place a stamp that is red." "Nothing felt and nothing seen, place a stamp that is green." "If there's mucus, wet and clear, place a baby white stamp here."

It is this method which is liberating the women of the world. Certainly pills and coils are dangerous and demeaning to women. For every ten women who are hospitalized because of the coil, there is only one hospitalized because of the pill. However, for every woman who dies because of the coil, there are ten who die because of the pill. In obstetrics the bottom line has become safety. In family planning the bottom line must become safety.

What loving husband and wife wants to armor themselves with condoms and diaphragms before participating in "total giving?"

This is the method which puts a woman in the driver's seat, but a couple won't go far unless the husband has a map of the road.

All couples are either trying to become pregnant or trying to avoid pregnancy. This method provides for both. Fertility awareness should be taught in every high school. There should be a Natural Family Planning Center in each town and a Natural Family Planning clinic in each hospital. A copy of this book should be in every home.

Dr. John J. Brennan, Assistant Clinical Professor (OB-GYN) Marquette Medical School; Diplomate American Board of Obstetrics and Gynaecology; Fellow of American College of Obstetrics and Gynaecology; Teaching staff of Milwaukee County General Hospital; President, National Federation of Catholic Physicians' Guilds, 1974; Chairman, National Commission for Human Life, Reproduction, and Rhythm, 1973–74; Medical Director, Human Life Foundation Project, U.S. Department of Health, Education and Welfare, 1974–75; Legislative Committee, Milwaukee County Medical Society, 1974; Board of Directors, National Federation of Natural Family Planning, 1974–76; Merit Award, Marquette University, 1973.

JOHN J. BRENNAN

Appendix 1

*THIS REPORT IS TAKEN IN PART FROM THE WORLD HEALTH ORGANIZA-
TION–SPECIAL PROGRAMME OF RESEARCH, DEVELOPMENT AND RE-
SEARCH TRAINING IN HUMAN REPRODUCTION.*
Seventh Annual Report, November 1978 (Unpublished Document).

RESEARCH

1. *Assessment of the Ovulation Method of natural family planning*

There are two basic problems relating to the use of NFP, i.e., the accurate identification of the fertile days of the menstrual cycle and implementing the abstinence required on these days. Furthermore, there is debate on whether or not all women are capable of detecting the signs and symptoms associated with ovulation. Considering these points, and the fact that very little objective data was available on the effectiveness of the ovulation, in 1975 the Programme initiated a multicentred clinical evaluation of the ovulation method.

The specific aims of the ovulation method study are to determine the percentage of women who are capable of recognizing changes in cervical mucus during the menstrual cycle; to correlate those changes with an objective parameter of ovulation, namely progesterone (or pregnanediol) levels in a selected number of cycles; to correlate the ability of women to observe cervical mucus changes with their social and medical data; and to determine the use-effectiveness and the theoretical effectiveness of the method in women who are capable of detecting changes in the cervical mucus. Centres with prior experience with the ovulation method, and with qualified teachers, were invited to participate. The five centres are in Auckland (New Zealand), Bangalore (India), Dublin (Ireland), Manila (Phillipines), and San Miguel (El Salvador). One hundred and fifty to two hundred subjects per centre were recruited who had not previously used a cervical mucus method and who were of proven fertility. Only ovulating women with a history of regular menstrual cycles, who had successfully completed a 3–6 month training period, entered the effectiveness study (13 cycles).

870 women were recruited for the study. Catholics constituted 83% of all subjects. The largest percentage of subjects of other religions was 33%. Hindus in Bangalore and 12% Protestants in Auckland.

About 40% of the women had never previously used any method of fertility regulation, 40% had had experience with periodic abstinence, 17% with withdrawal, 17% with the condom and only 19% and 5% with oral contraceptives and IUDs respectively. However, there was wide variation between centres in the frequency with which couples had previously used fertility regulating methods. Forty-nine per cent of the couples indicated "religious reasons" as their prime motivation for using the ovulation method. "Dissatisfaction with other methods" and "recommendation of an ovulation method user" was the prime motivation in 28% and 16% of the subjects, respectively.

These results are very preliminary and may only be valid for the sample population that participated in the study. In the first cycle following instruction a mean of 93% of the subjects showed an interpretable mucus pattern, i.e. the mucus pattern charted by the subject allowed the teacher to conclude that the subject was identifying her "symptoms" correctly. Results of the second and third teaching cycles were similar. The subject's understanding of the method following the first completed cycle in the teaching phase was assessed by the teacher as "excellent" or "good" in 91% of the subjects and "poor" in 9%. These figures had increased to 95% and 97% assessed as "excellent" or "good" and decreased to 5% and 3% as "poor", in the second and third cycles, respectively.

Although it is intended to use the life table method of analysis to report pregnancy rates when the study is completed the following rates were obtained by using the modified Pearl formula. As of 1 October 1978, during the teaching phase of the study approximately 870 women contributed 2685 cycles of exposure and 40 pregnancies occurred, i.e., 19.4 pregnancies per 100 woman-years (23.5 Auckland, 12.5 Bangalore, 10.4 Dublin, 24.7 Manila, 33.7 San Miguel). However, only three of the pregnancies occurred under circumstances where the method definitely appeared to be used correctly. Thus, the theoretical effectiveness of the method is 98.5%. These figures are in agreement with the findings of other studies.

The majority of the pregnancies experienced so far appear to be the result of couples knowingly "taking a chance" during the fertile phase, despite the fact that during each follow-up interview they declared their continued interest in participating in the study and using the method during the next cycle to avoid pregnancy. It appears that almost all of the women entering the study could be taught to identify the mucus symptoms associated with ovulation, that the ovulation method enables women to detect the fertile days of the menstrual cycle and that *when abstinence is adhered to during the fertile phase* the method appears to be very effective in preventing pregnancy.

REFERENCE

World Health Organization–Special Programme of Research, Development and Research Training in Human Reproduction–Seventh Annual Report November 1978, (Unpublished Document).

Appendix 2
Cervical Mucus and Identification of the Fertile Phase of the Menstrual Cycle

Anna M. Flynn
University Department of Obstetrics and Gynaecology
The Maternity Hospital, Queen Elizabeth Medical Centre
Birmingham 15

and

S. S. Lynch
Department of Clinical Endocrinology
The Birmingham and Midland Hospital for Women
Sparkhill, Birmingham 11

SUMMARY

Nine healthy fertile women were studied during 29 menstrual cycles. A cervical mucus grading system, assessed by the patient and used in conjunction with basal body temperature, was correlated with plasma levels of luteinizing hormone (LH), oestradiol and plasma progesterone. The results show that a patient can be taught to predict the time of ovulation by observing the changes in the cervical mucus.

In a previous paper (Flynn and Bertrand, 1973), it was shown that an assessment of cycle cervical mucus, based on the cervical score of Insler *et al* (1970), was a reliable and relatively simple means of making an objective evaluation of ovarian function. It requires, however, daily examination by a medical worker. To be practically useful, a method mucus assessment should be simple, convenient, and capable of interpretation by the patient herself. This paper attempts to assess the ability of the fertile woman to recognize and interpret cyclical changes in her cervical mucus.

METHODS

Patients. The study was carried out in nine healthy female women volunteers whose ages ranged from 26 to 44 years and parity from 3 to 6. Their social status ranged from Grades I to V. All had at some time observed a mucus discharge during the menstrual cycle, but had never quantified or charted it. Three cycles were studied in each of seven patients and four cycles in the remaining two.

Hormone assays. All hormonal estimations were carried out on serum. Twenty ml samples of blood were taken from an arm vein and allowed to clot at room temperature. Serum was separated after centrifugation and stored at -20 °C until assayed. Samples from any one cycle were estimated in the same assay. A basal sample for luteinizing hormone (LH), oestradiol and progesterone was taken between day 4 and day 9. Further samples for LH and oestradiol were taken consecutively from the day the patient first observed cervical mucus until she estimated that she no longer had fertile type mucus. The number of samples taken at this time averaged seven per cycle and varied between day 6 and day 25.

A further specimen of blood for progesterone assay was taken approximately seven days after the maximum mucus grade (MMG). LH was estimated by a double antibody radioimmunoassay using the reagents described by Lynch and Shirley (1975). The standard MRC 69/104 was supplied by the Division of Biological Standards, London. The steroid hormones were measured by radioimmunoassays using ammonium sulphate precipitation for the separation of free and bound fractions. The anti-oestradiol serum was prepared against the 6-oxime derivative as described by Dean *et al* (1971) and the progesterone serum used was as described by Furr (1973).

Clinical estimations. The basal body temperature (BBT) was taken throughout the cycle, or at least on sufficient days to show a biphasic pattern. The patients were asked to wipe the vulva with toilet paper both before and after micturition and make a note of the mucus present. They were instructed to classify their cervical mucus according to the cervical mucus grading system outlined by Brown (1973) (see Table 1). The day on which the patient had the maximum amount of clear mucus was taken as the day of maximum mucus grading (MMG) and as her interpretation of the day of ovulation. Where equal scores occurred on two days, the second of these was taken as the maximum. The ovulation or fertile phase of the cycle was defined as the day when the mucus grade was 5 or more. The results were recorded on the temperature charts.

RESULTS

All of the patients completed three cycles and two completed a fourth cycle, making a total of 29 cycles studied. No planned or unplanned pregnancies occurred. In all cycles the day of ovulation was taken as that of the LH peak.

BBT. The BBT showed a biphasic pattern in 26 cycles. One patient omitted to take her temperature during two cycles, and in a further patient the number of readings was judged insufficient to allow interpretation. There was a significant rise in progesterone in these three cycles.

TABLE 1.   Cervical Mucus Grading

TYPE	GRADING	DESCRIPTION
	-1	Dry sensation
	Definite change	
	1	Not dry, nothing seen
Infertile	2	Yellow or white, minimal
	3	Yellow or white, sticky
Possibly fertile	4	Cloudy, becoming clearer, sticky
	Definite change	
	5	Thinner, more stretchy
Fertile	7	Stretchy, lubricative, clear (may be cloudy)
	9	Wet, slippery, variable amount

Hormonal estimations. An LH peak was observed in all 29 cycles, ranging from 10 to 59 U/l. These values were 3 to 36 times the mean follicular LH levels. In all 29 cycles the basal levels of progesterone were less than 9 nmol/l. In 23 of the cycles the luteal levels were greater than 14 nmol/l and ranged from 15 to 72 nmol/l. Of the remaining six cycles, progesterone was not estimated in five of them until between days 25 and 28 of the cycle and the level ranged from 2 to 11 nmol/l, and in one cycle the sample was lost. However, there was a biphasic pattern in the BBT in these six cycles. The basal level of oestrogen ranged from 40 to 762 pmol/l, and in all cycles showed a preovulatory peak, with levels ranging from 541 to 2917 pmol/l. The oestrogen peak either preceded or coincided with the LH peak. In one patient a second oestrogen peak, higher than the estimated ovulation peak, occurred four days after the first oestrogen peak and three days after the LH peak. This second oestrogen peak coincided with a serum progesterone level of 27 nmol/l and was not reflected in the cervical mucus which was scored as 2.

Cervical mucus. All patients identified cervical mucus in all cycles but classification became easier with continued observation. The presence of seminal fluid after coitus caused some confusion during earlier cycles. One patient had a monilial infection of the vagina in the second half of the cycle; the infection was successfully treated and she charted her cervical mucus correctly in the preovulatory phases. The relationship between the day of MMG and the oestrogen or LH peaks is shown in Table II. The intervals between the first and the last day on which a fertile-type mucus (score 5 to 9) was noted and its relationship to other events in the menstrual cycle are shown in Table III, while Table IV gives the same information about 'any' type of mucus.

TABLE 2. Relationship Between MMG and Oestrogen or LH Peaks

	TIMING OF MMG RELATIVE TO	
NO. OF DAYS	OESTROGEN PEAK	LH PEAK
2 days before	0	3
1 day before	4	10
Same day	11	13
1 day after	12	3
2 days after	2	0
Mean value (days)	+0·41	−0·45

Except in the last line of the table, all figures indicate the number of patients in each group.

DISCUSSION

Our patients succeeded in identifying the fertile phase of the menstrual cycle by distinguishing the colour consistency and amount of cervical mucus present, and giving it a score (Table 1). Such a simple method, capable of accurate assessment and interpretation by the patient, enables the infertile woman to recognize whether or not she is ovulating, and if ovulating to plan intercourse at the time of her maximum fertility. This could avoid lengthy, inconvenient and expensive hormone profile studies.

TABLE 3.   Relationship Between the First and Last Days of Fertile Mucus (Score 5 or More) and Other Events in the Menstrual Cycle

NO. OF DAYS	INTERVAL BETWEEN LH PEAK AND		INTERVAL BETWEEN MMG AND	
	FIRST DAY OF FERTILE MUCUS	LAST DAY OF FERTILE MUCUS	FIRST DAY OF FERTILE MUCUS	LAST DAY OF FERTILE MUCUS
5	5	0	1	0
4	12	0	7	1
3	4	0	13	0
2	8	4	8	7
1	0	13	0	16
0	0	12	0	5
Mean value (days)	3·5	0·7	3·0	1·2

Except in the last line of the table, all figures indicate the number of patients in each group.

A natural family planning method must be able to detect impending ovulation at least 72 hours in advance, and subsequently identify the ovulatory event. In 8 of the 29 cycles studied (five patients) there was only a two-day preovulatory fertile mucus phase. However, the appearance of any mucus occurred on average 5·2 days before the LH peak, which agrees exactly with the findings of Billings et al (1972). It also appeared at least three days before both the LH peak and the MMG and this therefore might serve as a method of assessing the times of the cycle during which sexual abstinence should be observed in order to avoid a pregnancy. We found that social status was of no great importance in teaching a woman to recognize and chart the cervical mucus. Indeed, those of lower social grades seemed relatively more observant and more easily taught.

TABLE 4.   Relationship Between the First and Last Days of "Any" Mucus and Other Events in the Menstrual Cycle

NO. OF DAYS	INTERVAL BETWEEN LH PEAK AND		INTERVAL BETWEEN MMG AND	
	FIRST DAY OF "ANY" MUCUS	LAST DAY OF "ANY" MUCUS	FIRST DAY OF "ANY" MUCUS	LAST DAY OF "ANY" MUCUS
8-12	2	6	1	7
7	3	2	2	1
6	4	1	5	3
5	11	4	6	0
4	7	2	12	9
3	2	5	3	5
2	0	9	0	4
Mean value (days)	5·2	4·8	4·8	5·2

Except in the last line of the table, all figures indicate the number of patients in each group.

ACKNOWLEDGMENTS

We are indebted to the Catholic Marriage Advisory Council of England and Wales, through whose auspices we recruited our volunteers and who contributed financially through its Family Research Fund. We thank Professor W. R. Butt for his advice and encouragement throughout the course of the work; and the staff of the Department of Clinical Endocrinology. The Birmingham and Midland Hospital for Women, who carried out the hormone assays. Finally, our sincere thanks go to the patients who volunteered for this study.

REFERENCES

Billings, E.L., Billings, J. J., Brown, J. B., and Binger, H. G. (1972): *Lancet.* 1, 282.

Brown, J. B. (1973): *Ovulation Method Workshop.* Responsible Parenthood Association, Sydney, New South Wales. p 18.

Dean, P. D. G., Exley, D., and Johnson, M. W. (1971): *Steroids.* 18, 593.

Flynn, A. M., and Bertrand, P. V. (1973): *Journal of Obstetrics and Gynaecology of the British Commonwealth.* 80 152.

Furr, B. J. A. (1973): *Actu endocrinologica.* 72, 89.

Insler, V., Melmed, H., Eden, E., Serr, D., and Lunenfeld, B. (1970): *Clinical Application of Human Gonadotrophins.* Proceedings of a Workshop Conference, Hamburg 1970. Edited by G. Bettendorf and V. Insler. Georg Thieme Verlag, Stuttgart, p 87.

Lynch, S. S., and Shirley, A. (1975): *Journal of Endocrinology.* 65, 127.

Appendix 3
Rural Victoria
M. Ball

Author gives permission to reprint this appendix provided it is prefaced by the following paragraph:
"This trial is evidence of user-effectiveness of the "ovulation method" in a group of highly motivated couples. Each woman was instructed by a trained teacher and was well able to identify her own symptoms of ovulation, before entering the trial."

SUMMARY

124 couples were recruited between May 1973 and July 1974 for a prospective study of the effectiveness of observation of the cervical mucus (the "Ovulation Method") as a means of avoiding conception. Two couples were lost to follow up; the remainder contributed 1626 cycles of observation and experienced 21 unplanned pregnancies. This gives an overall unplanned pregnancy rate of 15.5 per 100 women years.

INTRODUCTION

It has long been known that the hormonal changes associated with ovulation often cause symptoms. Pain, slight vaginal bleeding, and change in the amount and appearance of cervical mucus are most commonly encountered, of which the last has received most attention. In a cycle of 28 days the days following the cessation of menses are marked by an absence of mucus, accompanied by a sensation of 'dryness'. These are followed by a variable number of days in which mucus, which is at first cloudy and sticky, appears. As the time of ovulation approaches the mucus becomes stretchy and slippery, accompanied by a sensation of 'wetness'. After ovulation the mucus ceases or changes to a sticky type and the sensation of wetness is no longer present. The last day of any observation of wetness is known as Peak. Billings, Billings, Brown and Burger[1] have shown that the peak mucus change correlates closely with the time of ovulation as assessed by measurement of plasma luteinising hormone and urinary oestrogen and pregnanediol; the peak mucus occurred not earlier than three days before and not later than two days after the day of ovulation in 22 women whom they studied.

A number of authors have recommended that the change in mucus be used to determine the day of ovulation in order to avoid coitus at the fertile time in an attempt to regulate births. Billings[1,2] in particular has strongly recommended this method. The first prospective field trial of the method was however not reported until 1972.[3] This method concerned 282 couples in the island of Tonga who used the method through 2593 cycles. The authors calculated a failure rate from 3 unplanned pregnancies, excluding another 50 when couples had stated that they had "taken a chance" by having intercourse when they knew mucus was present. The Pearl formula applied to these 3 pregnancies is 1.4 per 100 women years: applied to the 53 pregnancies it is 25 per 100 women years.

The present study includes as unplanned those pregnancies resulting from 'risk taking' but tables them separately to enable easier comparison with other studies.

METHOD

The survey involved 124 women, aged 20–39 years inclusive, who contributed 1635 cycles. All had carried at least one pregnancy to term and had observed at least one ovulatory cycle since the last birth. The participants were recruited from Natural Family Planning Centres throughout Australia where they had received personal instruction from trained female instructors and from whom they received record charts and coloured stamps to mark the different phases of the menstrual cycle. The days of observation of mucus symptoms were marked on the chart with white stamps bearing the picture of a baby, thus producing a visual aid to recognition of fertility. In teaching the method great emphasis was placed on the need for good communication between husband and wife.

The clients sent their charts, at the end of each cycle, to the study centre. If, after two cycles, a chart had not been received a reminder was sent with further reminders if necessary. By this means only two women were lost to follow up, leaving 122 who contributed a total of 1626 cycles. The protocol required that intercourse in the pre-ovulatory phase should only take place if the woman observed a sensation of dryness, no mucus of any type being present; these days were recorded with a plain green stamp. Because the presence of seminal fluid the day following intercourse may make observation difficult, the rule was that the day following intercourse should always be considered "not dry".

Intercourse in the post-ovulatory phase was allowed when the client had recorded four consecutive days from the peak symptom; peak being described as the last day of any "fertile-type" mucus or wet sensation.

After the study had begun, some centres began to allow clients to use days in the pre-ovulatory phase when "sticky, cloudy mucus" was present.[4] A number of survey participants took advantage of this despite the protocol. Days of unchanging "sticky, cloudy mucus" were recorded with a plain yellow stamp.

RESULTS

The age distribution of the clients was: 20–24 years, 3; 25–29 years, 29; 30–34 years, 65; 35–39 years, 27. The parity was: 3 had 1 child, 16 had 2, 35 had 3, 34 had 4, 19 had 5, 9 had 6, 3 had 7, 3 had 8, 2 had 9. The outcome is shown in Table 1.

TABLE 1.   Outcome

WITHDRAWN BECAUSE		NO. OF CLIENTS
Planning a baby		5
Unplanned pregnancy		21
Contraception no longer needed		4
Changed to other method		8
Contraception abandoned though needed		2
Moved away		2
Lost to follow up		2
	Total	124

Among the 21 pregnancies in 4 the client had, as far as could be ascertained, followed the instructions given in the protocol; in 8 cases she had not and in 9 she had used days in the pre-ovulatory phase when "sticky, cloudy mucus" was present which was not allowed by the protocol but was subsequently introduced in some of the centres. The total unplanned pregnancy rate per 100 women years according to the Pearl formula is 15.5. The proportions attributable to the users taking a known risk and to the use of pre-ovulatory days in which sticky cloudy mucus was present are given in Table 2.

TABLE 2.   Unplanned Pregnancy Rate in. Various Groups

User took conscious risk	6.7
Used pre-ovulatory days with "sticky cloudy mucus"	5.9
Intercourse on "dry days" only	2.9
Total unplanned pregnancy rate	15.5

DISCUSSION

The protocol was designed to study the effectiveness of the use of the pre- and post-ovulatory phases of the cycle as determined by the cervical mucus symptom as a means of avoiding conception. The survey showed an overall unplanned pregnancy rate of 15.5 per 100 women years. Only four pregnancies occurred to couples who confined intercourse to the pre-ovulatory dry days and to the post-ovulatory days from the fourth day after the peak symptom giving a biological failure rate of 2.9 pregnancies per 100 women years.

Couples who used days of "sticky, cloudy" pre-ovulatory mucus as well as pre-ovulatory dry days and days from fourth day after the peak symptom produced nine pregnancies. The introduction of the teaching that the pre-ovulatory days when "sticky cloudy" mucus was present could be marked with a yellow stamp and used for intercourse created difficulties as this teaching was not envisaged when the protocol for the survey was planned. The literature published with the introduction of the yellow stamp[4] advocated the use of pre-ovulatory "sticky, cloudy" mucus only in certain circumstances. It was decided that any survey participant following this teaching should be left in the survey but be the subject of a separate category. Couples who took a conscious risk produced 8 pregnancies; in each case the woman had recorded the day used as fertile and had recorded with the visual aid of a "baby stamp."

The results of this study may be compared with those achieved in prospective studies of other natural methods of conception control.

The report by Marshall[5] of a study of the combined calendar/temperature method for couples using both the pre-ovulatory and post-ovulatory phases of the cycle showed an overall pregnancy rate of 19.3 per 100 women years. The "ovulation method" achieved a better effectiveness rate than the calendar/temperature method provided that intercourse in the pre-ovulatory phase was confined to dry days only.

In a study of the temperature method where intercourse was confined to the post-ovulatory phase alone, Marshall[5] showed a pregnancy rate of 6.6 pregnancies per 100 women years. No valid comparison can be made beween this result and the "ovulation method" as used in the present survey because there was no group in which the couples confined intercourse to the post-ovulatory phase of the cycle.

ACKNOWLEDGMENTS

I would like to thank the clients and the instructors for their co-operation, Mrs. Nola Burns for secretarial assistance, Professor John Marshall for advice on the design of the trial and the Family Research Trust for financial support.

REFERENCES

1. Billings, E. L., Billings, J. J., Brown, J. B., and Burger, H. G. Lancet 1972, 1, 282
2. Billings, J. J. The Ovulation Method. The Advocate Press, Melbourne, 1964.
3. Weissman, M. C., Foliaki, F., Billings, E. L., and Billings, J. J. Lancet 1972, 2, 813.
4. Billings, E. L., Billings, J. J. and Catarinich, M. The Atlas of The Ovulation Method. The Advocate Press, Melbourne, 1973.
5. Marshall, J. Lancet 1968, 2, 8.

Appendix 4
Symptoms and Hormonal Changes Accompanying Ovulation

E. L. Billings
J. J. Billings
J. B. Brown
H. G. Burger

Medical Research Centre, Prince Henry's Hospital, Melbourne; Melbourne University Department of Obstetrics and Gynaecology, Royal Women's Hospital, Melbourne; and Catholic Family Planning Centre, Melbourne, Victoria, Australia

SUMMARY

To determine whether normal women could predict and identify symptomatically the occurrence of ovulation, twenty-two volunteers were instructed in a pattern of vaginal "mucus symptoms" which had been established previously. Plasma luteinising hormone and urinary oestrogens and pregnanediol were measured to provide a "hormonal estimate" of the day of ovulation. A characteristic "lubricative" mucus identified by all the women occurred on the day of ovulation in five, 1 day before in nine, and 2 days before in four. The onset of mucus symptoms occurred 6·2 days (mean) before ovulation. It is concluded that the time of ovulation can be identified clinically, without recourse to temperature measurement or more specialised tests.

INTRODUCTION

The ability of a woman to predict and identify the time of ovulation, by means of her own symptoms, would have obvious applications in fertility control and in the management of infertility. "Natural" methods of family planning are usually based on a calendar record[1,2] of past menstrual cycles (the "rhythm method"), from which the fertile time of the cycle can be calculated, or on a basal body temperature (B.B.T) record,[3,4] from which the occurrence of ovulation can be judged retrospectively, or a combination of the two. The rhythm method is restrictive in that it must take account of the woman's longest and shortest recorded cycle; the B.B.T. method lacks specificity, and does not identify ovulation prospectively.

TABLE 1.   Analysis of Hormonal and Symptomatic Indices of Ovulation

SUBJECT	CYCLE LENGTH	DAY OF LH PEAK (PLASMA)	DAY OF TOTAL OES-TROGEN PEAK (URINE)	DAY OF SIGNIFICANT RISE IN PREGNAN-EDIOL (URINE)	DAY OF PEAK SYMPTOM	HORMO-NAL ESTI-MATE OF OVULA-TION (DAYS)	DAY OF FIRST RECORDED SYMPTOM	DAY OF RISE IN B.B.T.
1	30	16	15	. .	16	17	10	18
2	28	14	14	. .	14	15	11	16
3	35	. .	24	. .	23	25	16	24
4	25	14	13	15	16	15	11	4
5	27	12	11	13	11	13	6	13
6	25	13	13	16	12	14	9	14
7	25	13	13	16	12	14	7	14
8	28	13	12	18	13	14	6	15
9	27	15	15	18	13	16	8	?16*
10	33	. .	19	20	17	20	11	23
11	22	10	9	12	11	11	8	12
12	29	14	14	16	14	15	11	16
13	26	14	12	12	11	12 (15)	9	14
14	27	11	10	12	12	12	9	14
15	26	11	10	12	12	12	7	13
16	25	12	12	13	12	13	7	16
17	27	13	13	13	13	14	5	15
18	28	15	14	16	14	16	7	17
19	31	17	17	17	18	18	10	19
20	25	11	11	13	12	12	6	14
21	27	11	10	13	14	12	9	13
22	33	19	20	20	19	20	10	22

. . Sample collected at inappropriate part of cycle.
* Unsatisfactory B.B.T. record.

We have found that women can be taught to recognise a pattern of vaginal mucous discharge which occurs at about the time of ovulation, that there is a close correlation between those symptoms and the day of ovulation as estimated from hormone-excretion patterns, and that impending ovulation can be predicted for a period long enough to be of practical use for fertility control. The clinical application of the combination of symptoms and changes in B.B.T. has been described previously[5] as the "ovulation method".

METHODS

Symptoms of Ovulation

In the past fifteen years two of us (E. L. B. and J. J. B.) have interviewed several hundred women to define the mucous-discharge pattern occurring at the periovulatory period of the menstrual cycle. The major features of these symptoms are as follows:

(a) Menstrual bleeding is followed by a variable number of days on which no vaginal loss is present ("dry days").

(b) The onset of the "mucus symptoms" is characterised by the appearance of increasing quantities of "cloudy" or "sticky" secretion; the duration of this phase is variable (see below).

(c) This is followed by the occurrence of clear, slippery, lubricative mucus, having the physical characteristics of raw white of egg *(Spinnbarkeit)*; this has been termed the "peak symptom". It characteristically lasts for 1–2 days, and the last day of its occurrence is referred to as the day of the peak symptom in the results presented.

(d) The "peak symptom" is followed by the presence of thick, "tacky", opaque mucus, the duration of which is variable.

Women Studied

Twenty-two women attending the Catholic Family Planning Centre, Melbourne, were chosen for the study solely because of their willingness to cooperate, and the series studied is a consecutive one. Several were unconvinced, after initial instruction, that they could readily identify mucus symptoms, but all were well motivated to assist in the investigation. All were married, their ages ranged from 25 to 42 years, and they were of proven fertility (1–7 children; modal number, 2). Menstrual cycle lengths varied from 22 to 35 days, mean 27·6. Each woman was asked to keep a daily record of her mucus symptoms, and to measure vaginal B.B.T. before rising in the morning. Serial daily blood-samples were collected on 9–10 consecutive days around the expected time of midcycle and urine collections (24-hour) were made throughout the cycle in all except the first six women, who collected only at midcycle. The blood was collected by venepuncture, by a nurse visiting the home. The women were, therefore, normal volunteer housewives of proven fertility, studied in their own homes.

Hormone Assays

Luteinising hormone (L.H.) was measured by a solid phase radioimmunoassay similar to that previously described[6] for human growth hormone, using radioiodinated human L.H. (donated by Dr. A. Stockell Hartree), and anti-L.H. antiserum. Results were expressed as m.I.U. per ml., using a laboratory standard of pituitary gonadotrophin which had been characterised biologically in terms of the second international reference preparation of human menopausal gonadotrophins (L.H. activity,[7] 144 I.U.. per mg.). Total urinary oestrogens[8] and pregnanediol[9] were measured by previously published methods.

Hormonal Estimate of Day of Ovulation

The midcycle peak of plasma-L.H. occurs about 16 hours before ovulation, as judged by biopsy of the corpus luteum,[10] and the midcycle peak of urinary oestrogen excretion usually occurs on the day before the plasma-L.H. peak or on the same day.[11] Urinary pregnanediol excretion rises with the establishment of luteal function.

We defined the day of ovulation as the day after the midcycle plasma-L.H. peak; this usually corresponded to the day on which urinary pregnanediol excretion had reached a value more than twice the mean follicular-phase level. With one exception, the peak of urinary oestrogen excretion occurred 0–2 days before the estimated day of ovulation. In two women (nos. 3 and 10), it was clear that blood-samples had not been obtained at midcycle (cycle lengths were 35 and 33 days, respectively), and the day of ovulation was assumed to be the day after the total oestrogen peak, confirmed by a pregnanediol rise in subject no. 10.

B.B.T. Rise

For each woman, a line was drawn on the B.B.T. chart ("the marginal line"),[5] below which the temperatures in the late follicular phase were found, and above which the temperature had reached luteal-phase levels. The first day on which the temperature lay above the marginal line was termed the day of rise in B.B.T.

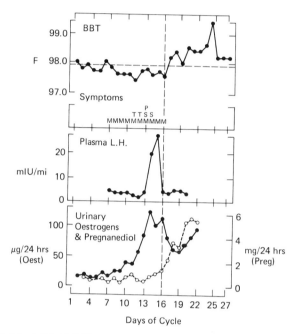

Subject 18: B.B.T., mucus symptoms, plasma-L.H., and urinary oestrogens and pregnanediol.

Symptoms are characterised as mucus (M), tacky mucus (TM), slippery or lubricative mucus (SM), and P (pain). M indicates maximum quantity of mucus; the day of the peak symptom was taken as the second day marked SM. The vertical dotted line indicates the day of ovulation estimated hormonally. The horizontal dotted line on the B.B.T. record is the "marginal line".

RESULTS

The results are summarised in tables I and II, and a typical cycle is shown in the figure. In subject no. 9, peak excretion of pregnanediol in the luteal phase reached only 1·1 mg. per 24 hours, suggesting that a fully functioning corpus luteum was not established; there was, however, a clear peak in urinary oestrogen excretion and in plasma-L.H. (23·5 m.I.U. per ml.). In subject no. 13 there were inconsistencies in the hormonal measurements; thus, although there was a peak in plasma-L.H. (10·6 m.I.U. per ml.) on day 14, urinary pregnanediol had increased significantly on day 12; the day of ovulation in this subject was taken as day 12 or possibly day 15 (although on day 15 pregnanediol was already 5·6 mg. per 24 hours).

Table II shows that ovulation, as assessed hormonally, occurred 0·9 days (mean) after the occurrence of the peak symptom, with a range from 3 days after to 2 days before (in one subject). Furthermore, the mean interval from the onset of mucus symptom to ovulation was 6·2 days, with a range from 3 to 10 days. The rise in B.B.T. generally occurred 1–2 days after ovulation.

TABLE 2. Correspondence Between Day of Ovulation as Estimated from Symptoms and Hormonal Measurements: Interval from Onset of Symptoms to Ovulation

SUBJECT	INTERVAL: PEAK SYMPTOM TO DAY OF OVULATION (DAYS)	INTERVAL: FIRST RECORDED SYMPTOM TO DAY OF OVULATION (DAYS)
1	1	7
2	1	4
3	2	9
4	−1	4
5	2	7
6	1	4
7	2	7
8	1	8
9	3	8
10	3	9
11	0	3
12	1	4
13	1(4)	3(6)
14	0	3
15	0	5
16	1	6
17	1	9
18	2	9
19	0	8
20	0	6
21	−2	3
22	1	10
mean	0·9	6·2

DISCUSSION

We have found that twenty-two normal housewives, selected only because they were willing to participate in the study, could be taught to recognise a pattern of vaginal mucous secretion during the menstrual cycle, and to distinguish the occurrence of a particular symptom—namely, lubricative clear mucus. This "peak symptom" was closely correlated with the day of ovulation, as estimated from measurements of plasma-L.H. and urinary total oestrogens and pregnanediol. Furthermore, the mucus symptoms began, on average, 6·2 days before the putative occurrence of ovulation, thus providing a useful indication of impending ovulation. The peak symptom was closely associated with the peak of urinary oestrogen excretion, which is consistent with the effects of oestrogen on the cervical mucus glands.

These observations provide a basis for a method of birth regulation which depends solely on observations which can be made by most normal women, and on the avoidance of sexual intercourse from the time of onset of these symptoms until after the occurrence of the peak symptom. Such a method (the "ovulation method") is now being studied; women are instructed to abstain from intercourse at the onset of the mucus symptoms, and sexual activity may be resumed on the fourth day after the "peak symptom". Furthermore, a couple who are having difficulty in conceiving can be instructed to concentrate their efforts on the days of the "peak symptom".

The widespread application of such a method clearly requires confirmation of its reliability in practice; in addition, it demands that women be taught to recognise their symptoms, and thus its applicability to all classes in society must be demonstrated. Such studies are in progress.

Our findings have also proved useful in physiological studies of the hormonal events which surround ovulation. A World Health Organisation list[12] of research needs in fertility control by periodic abstinence included "a formula that may give a better estimate of the time of ovulation than the current formulae" and "simple tests for the accurate prediction of ovulation". Our results suggest that these needs may be met by simple clinical means.

This study was supported by three anonymous donations through St. Vincent's Hospital, Melbourne, and by grants from the National Health and Medical Research Council. The co-operation of Rev. F. Richards and the medical staff of the Catholic Family Planning Centre is gratefully acknowledged. Sister McLennan collected the blood-samples; technical assistance was provided by Mrs. M. Wajnstok, Mrs. C. Reichman, Mrs. L. Parker, Miss G. de Haan, Miss J. McLaughlin, and Miss J. Sedgman. Miss C. Freestone drew the figure and Mrs. J. Volfsbergs typed the manuscript.

Requests for reprints should be addressed to H. G. B., Medical Research Centre, Prince Henry's Hospital, St. Kilda Road, Melbourne, Victoria 3004, Australia.

REFERENCES

1. Ogino, K. *Zbl. Gynäk*, 1930, 54, 464.
2. Knaus, H. *ibid.* 1929, 53, 2192.
3. Ferin, J. *Brux. méd.* 1947, 27, 2786.
4. Marshall, J. *Lancet*, 1968, ii, 8.
5. Billings, J. J. The Ovulation Method. Melbourne, 1971.
6. Catt, K. J., Tregear, G. W., Burger, H. G., Skermer, C. *Clinica chim. Acta*, 1970, 27, 267.
7. Parlow, A. F. *in* Human Pituitary Gonadotrophins: A Workshop Conference (edited by A. Albert); p. 301. Springfield, Illinois, 1971.
8. Brown, J. B., MacLeod, S. C., Macnaughton, C., Smith, M. A., Smyth, B. *F. Endocr.* 1968, 42, 5.
9. Barrett, S. A., Brown, J. B. *ibid.* 1970, 47, 471.
10. Yussman, M. A., Taymor, M. L. *F. clin. Endocr. Metab.* 1970, 30, 396.
11. Burger, H. G. Catt, K. J., Brown, J. B. *ibid.* 1968, 28, 1508.
12. *Wld Hlth Org. tech. Rep. Ser.* 1967, no. 360.

Appendix 5

Use-Effectiveness and Analysis of Satisfaction Levels with the Billings Ovulation Method: Two-Year Pilot Study * †

Hanna Klaus, M.D.‡
Joan Goebel, M.D.§
Ralph E. Woods, M.D.¶
Mary Castles, Ph.D.‖
George Zimny, Ph.D.#

Department of Gynecology and Obstetrics and Department of Human Behavior, School of Medicine, and Department of Research Methodology, School of Nursing and Allied Health, St. Louis University, St. Louis, Missouri 63104

A 2-year study of 135 women using the Billings Ovulation Method as their method of family planning is reported. There were 1381 exposure cycles during the 1st year and 580 during the 2nd year. The total conception rates were 1.303 for the 1st year and 1.896 for the 2nd year. If one subtracts the user failures from these rates, the biologic failure rates are 0.072 for the 1st year and 0.517 for the 2nd year. The continuation rate is 51.8%. An analysis of satisfaction levels is presented with a discussion of possible underlying emotional factors.

*Received November 30, 1976; revised April 22, 1977, and June 6, 1977; accepted June 7, 1977.

* Performed as a volunteer project by the authors; there was no commitment or funding on the part of St. Louis University.

† Presented in part at the Eighth World Congress of Obstetrics and Gynecology, October 19, 1976, Mexico City, Mexico.

‡ Department of Gynecology and Obstetrics, School of Medicine. Present address and address for reprint requests: Hanna Klaus, M.D., Director, Department of Obstetrics and Gynecology, St. Francis Hospital, 929 North St. Francis, Wichita, Kan. 67214.

§ Clinical Faculty. Presently retired.

¶ Department of Gynecology and Obstetrics, School of Medicine.

‖ Department of Research Methodology, School of Nursing and Allied Health. Present address: Wayne State University, Detroit, Mich.

Department of Human Behavior, School of Medicine.

This is the report of a pilot project utilizing 135 women who used the Billings Ovulation Method[1] during the study period September 1, 1973, to August 31, 1975. A portion of this study has been reported as the 1st-year pilot project.[2]

The Billings Ovulation Method is the most recent arrival in the area of natural family planning. It is a predictive method which is based on the development of a changing mucus symptom. The appearance of mucus has been shown to correlate with the rising estrogen level generated by the developing follicle. The mucus reaches a peak of wetness which has been shown to correlate with the luteinizing hormone peak. Ovulation is hypothesized to occur from 9 hours before to 48 hours after the "peak symptom." Hence, all of the mucus days preceding the "peak symptom" plus the 72 hours following are presumed to be the fertile days of a woman.[1,3]

At the time the study was begun, use-effectiveness studies were sparse, hence validation of the hypothesis appeared important. This larger report carries forward the women of the 1st-year group and adds women who had begun to use the method before the 1st year of study ended (August 31, 1974) but whose charts were not then available for inclusion. In order to conform to the life-table method of use-effectiveness,[4] the entire 2-year sample was restudied statistically and arranged in ordinal months; hence the numbers in the 1st-year pilot project do not necessarily correspond to the present study.

MATERIALS AND METHODS

The self-selected volunteer groups were instructed in the interpretation of their mucus signs according to the criteria of Billings et al.[1] and in recording these signs on a prepared chart. They also recorded acts of sexual intercourse and indicated the days on which these occurred. All acceptors had been evaluated in follow-up at least once and had brought a chart which could be interpreted by the authors. Acceptors are defined as those willing to commit themselves to the use of this method for fertility control and to provide information for the study. Of 630 persons instructed, 135 agreed to become acceptors. Age and reproductive and contraceptive histories were recorded, as well as menstrual and mucus cycles, acts of coitus, and any observation the subject offered. To show that the spectrum of individuals afforded a reasonably broad range of fertility potential, fecundable status, as defined in Table 1A, was recorded for each woman at the time of entry in the study (Table 2A). Classification by status as defined in Table 1B was recorded for each subject at termination (Table 2B). This approach follows methodology for recording as suggested by Tietze and Lewit[4] and was adopted because we were unable to provide matched study and control groups. Tables 2 and 3 show the social characteristics of the group. Table 4 lists concurrent and previous methods of contraception.

TABLE 1. Definitions of Fecundable and Terminal Statuses

A: FECUNDABLE STATUS (BEGINNING)	B: TERMINAL STATUS (ENDING)
S_0 Fecundable, not exposed	0 Using method (protected by method)
S_1 Fecundable, 1st interval (exposure to 1st conception)	1 Lost to follow-up (if no response to mail or phone calls)
S_2 Fecundable, 2nd interval (delivery to 2nd conception)	2 Discontinuation–unable to identify mucus cycle
S_3 Fecundable, 3rd interval	3 Discontinuation–unable to use method (personal)
S_4 S_5, S_6 (interval)	4 Discontinuation–unable to use method (medical)
S_7 Fecundable, postpartum (exclude 3 mo if not lactating, 6 mo if lactating)	5 Discontinuation–no need for further protection
	6 Discontinuation–continued exposure to conception
S_8 Fecundable, postabortion (exclude 6 wk after event)	7 Discontinuation–change of method
S_9 Lactating >6 mo	8 Discontinuation–no desire for protection (planning pregnancy)
	9 Discontinuation–accidental pregnancy, biologic failure
	10 Discontinuation–pregnant, but plan to continue method after pregnancy
	11 Discontinuation–accidental pregnancy, personal failure

TABLE 2. Fecundable and Terminal Statuses of Acceptors by Age Group[a]

A: FECUNDABLE STATUS (BEGINNINGS)

AGE	NO.	%	1	2	3	4	5	6	7	8	9
18	0	0.000	0	0	0	0	0	0	0	0	0
18–24	23	17.037	19	1	0	1	1	1	0	0	0
25–29	35	25.925	9	4	11	5	2	1	2	0	1
30–34	40	29.629	1	3	4	7	8	10	6	1	0
35–39	22	16.296	0	1	4	6	3	8	0	0	0
40–44	14	10.370	0	0	2	1	1	10	0	0	0
>45	1	0.740	0	0	0	0	0	1	0	0	0
Total	135		29	9	21	20	15	31	8	1	1

B: TERMINAL STATUS (ENDINGS)

00	01	02	03	04	05	06	07	08	09	10	11
0	0	0	0	0	0	0	0	0	0	0	0
11	5	0	1	0	1	0	0	3	0	1	0
5	6	1	4	0	1	0	2	11	1	4	0
25	3	0	5	0	0	1	3	1	1	1	0
16	0	0	1	0	0	0	1	3	0	1	0
12	0	0	1	0	0	0	0	0	0	1	0
1	0	0	0	0	0	0	0	0	0	0	0
70	14	1	12	0	2	1	7	18	2	8	0

[a] At the beginning of the study, all subjects were in terminal status 00, so those totals correspond with the regular age breakdown.

TABLE 3.   Residential and Educational Characteristics of Acceptors

	EDUCATION					
RESIDENCE	PRIMARY	SECONDARY	SECONDARY[+]	PROFESSIONAL	NO RESPONSE	TOTAL
Rural	0	1	3	0	0	4
Urban	0	37	59	26	3	125
No response	0	0	0	0	6	6
Total		38	62	26	9	135

When the charts were reviewed for follow-up at the conclusion of the 2nd year of study, all subjects were asked in person, by telephone, or by letter whether they were still using the method, whether they were using the method to avoid or to achieve pregnancy, and whether they were satisfied with their use of the method. Their replies were recorded verbatim and assigned a value of 1 (low) to 5 (high) on a satisfaction level. They were also asked whether they were still charting on the prepared chart or, if not, how they were recording.

TABLE 4.   Concurrent and Previous Contraceptive Methods

CONCURRENT METHOD		PREVIOUS METHOD	
CONTRACEPTIVE	NO. OF WOMEN	CONTRACEPTIVE	NO. OF WOMEN
Condom	10	Condom	15
Withdrawal	1	Withdrawal	10
Temperature-rhythm	16	Temperature-rhythm	53
Calendar-rhythm	1	Calendar-rhythm	48
Hormones[a]	3	Hormones	57
Jelly or foam	2	Hormones >6 mo previously[b]	40
		Jelly or foam	12
		Diaphragm	5
		Intrauterine device	7
		None	20
		Total	267[c]

[a] Estrogen or progesterone given for regulation of menstrual cycle.
[b] As the cycle often requires 6 months to return to normal after discontinuation of hormonal contraception, the distinction is made.
[c] Many reported many previous methods.

RESULTS

The subjects' entries, exits, and fecundable and terminal statuses were analyzed by the life-table method.[4] The results are given in Table 5. Eighteen couples had used the method to try to achieve pregnancy. By the close of the study, four couples had succeeded.

**TABLE 5. Unplanned Pregnancies Resulting from Personal
(T-11) and Biologic (T-9) Failure**

DURATION OF USE	NO. OF EXPOSURES	NO. OF PREGNANCIES T-11	NO. OF PREGNANCIES T-9	CONCEPTION RATES T-11		CONCEPTION RATES T-9	
mo							
6	760	7	0	0.921	1.231	0.000	0.072
12	621	10	1	1.610		0.161	
18	413	6	1	1.453		0.242	
24	156	2	2	1.282	1.379	1.292	0.517
27	11	0	0	0.000		0.000	

Table 6 is a histogram which compares graphically the personal (group 2, T-11) and biologic (group 1, T-9) failures. Group 2 comprised 25 subjects, while group 1 numbered 4. A comparison of group 1 (biologic failure) with group 2 (personal failure) by the log-rank method of Azen et al.[5] yielded the following data ($N=$ 29 subjects):

GROUP	NO. OF PATIENTS	OBSERVED PREGNANCIES (O)	EXPECTED PREGNANCIES (E)	O/E
1	4	1	2.99	0.33
2	25	18	16.01	1.12
		Over-all $\chi^2 = 1.78$ on 1 DF:$P = 0.1816$		

The χ^2 value of 1.78 and the P value of 0.1816 indicate that the statistic tends to be non-significant.

Analysis of the satisfaction levels revealed values of 3.8 for group 2 and 2.2 for group 1. The comparable satisfaction level for 55 T-O subjects (using the method to avoid pregnancy) = 4.4, whereas the level for the 18 women who were planning pregnancy (T-8) = 4.6. The remaining 19 women in discontinuation categories were classified as follows: T-3 (personal reasons) = 12, satisfaction level = 2.3; the other 7 were scattered in the remaining discontinuation categories (see Table 1B). A number of women had discontinued the use of the prepared chart and were recording on their kitchen calendars. Of our study group of 135 women, 69 submitted charts, 44 used calendars, and 22 relied on their memories. Although the charting was subjective, the study design precluded pelvic examination, which could have offered objective corroboration. Charting of acts of intercourse is necessarily subjective and depends on the cooperation of the subjects.

A comparison of results with other methods of family planning is shown in Table 7.

DISCUSSION

The numbers of this pilot project are not yet significant because the N is incomplete.

The present Billings Ovulation Method designates the beginning of the fertile time of a woman as the time of the first appearance of any vaginal mucus; the fertile period continues for a full 72 hours after the "peak symptom." The method, while still unrefined, is nonetheless completely physiologic.

TABLE 6.   Histographic Comparison of Groups 1 and 2.[a]

Probability	Probability of occurrence of unplanned pregnancy

```
1.000-  •••••••••]]1111111111111111111111111111111111111111111111111111111111111111111
        I        2                                                     1
        I        222222222                                             1
        I            2                                                 1
        I            2                                                 1
        I            222222222222222222222222222222                    1
        I                                2                             1
        I                                2                             1
        I                                2                             1
        I                                2                             1
0.800-  I                                2                             1
        I                                2                             1
        I                                222222222          1111111111111111111111111111111111111111
        I                                    2
        I                                    2
        I                                    2
        I                                    2
        I                                    2
        I                                    2
0.600-  I                                    222222222
        I                                        2
        I                                        222222222222222222
        I                                                        2
        I                                                        2
        I                                                        2
        I                                                        2
        I                                                        222222222
        I                                                            2
0.400-  I                                                            2
        I                                                            22222222222222222222
        I                                                                                2
        I                                                                                2
        I
        I
        I
        I
        I
0.200-  I
        I
        I
        I
        I
        I
        I
        I
        I
0.0  -  I-----------------------------------------------------------------------------------
        I                I                I                I                I                I
```

[a]Group 1, accidental pregnancy—biologic failure; group 2, accidental pregnancy—personal failure.

TABLE 7. Comparison of Use-Effectiveness and Continuation Rates by Life-Table Method and Pearl Formula

		USE-EFFECTIVENESS			
		LIFE-TABLE METHOD		PEARL FORMULA[a]	
REFERENCE	CONTRACEPTIVE	DURATION OF USE	PREGNANCIES 100 WOMEN-MO	PREGNANCIES 100 WOMAN-YR	CONTINUATION RATE
		mo			%
Tietze and Lewit[6]	Oral	6	3.9		75.50
		12	8.03		60.73
		18	13.9		49.70
Tietze and Lewit[6]	Intrauterine device	6	2.36		87.65
		12	4.63		78.4
		18	6.85		69.63
Rice et al[7]	Basal body temperature chart			8.14	
Rölzer[8]	Symptothermal method			0.68	
Lane et al[9]	Diaphragm and jelly	12	1.9–2.2		83.9–82.8
Dunn[10]	All natural family planning methods				
	Biologic failure			2.7	23.6[b]
	Personal failure			2.0	52.2[c]
	Total			4.7	
Present series (Table 5)	Ovulation Method				
	Biologic failure	12	0.072		51.8[b]
		24	0.517		
	Personal failure	12	1.231		13.0[c]
		24	1.379		
	Total	12	1.303		
		24	1.896		
Gupta et al[11]	Intrauterine device	12	0.3		66.8
		24	1.2		41.2
		36	1.7		20.3

[a] When authors reported data as pregnancies/100 woman-years their format was followed.
[b] To prevent pregnancy.
[c] Planning pregnancy.

No one undertakes an infertility investigation until the couple has had 1 year of unprotected coitus. Therefore, the figures begin to take on statistical significance only by the end of the 1st year, and become fully significant by the end of the 2nd year.[12] The life-table forms of data analysis are therefore more illuminating than the old Pearl formula, which often was based on extrapolations and did not necessarily include the events that occur during the period of reproductive life. The current approach of this pilot project affords a method of comparing data obtained from diverse methodologies of periodic abstinence.

The number of women for whom terminal statuses were available ($N = 135$) makes this pilot study worthy of note. Ten women in the 1st year study were lost to follow-up, whereas several who were continued into the 2nd calendar year did not complete the entire year for a number of reasons, as given in the discontinuation listing. The "surviving" users, with one exception, were willing to state their reasons for continuation or discontinuation. The one exception refused to talk in two attempted telephone interviews.

Some of our users, while in the terminal statuses given at the time of summation, have moved through intermediate statuses (for instance, terminal status 6). There were two women in this group who decided not to plan pregnancy but who did continue exposure to conception. Both became pregnant. At the end of the study year, they decided that they would now begin to use the method to prevent further pregnancy. As one of these women said, "Now I know the rules mean what they say."

The satisfaction levels for women who were using the method and were protected by it (T-0), for those planning pregnancy (T-8), and for those achieving it are understandable, but the relatively high satisfaction level of women who used fertile days while not planning pregnancy (T-11) is significant. One speculation is that, because they knew they were using fertile times, they decided to make the best of them. Another speculation is that their use of fertile days despite an initial intention to avoid pregnancy might represent an unconscious motivation for pregnancy stronger than a conscious motivation for pregnancy avoidance. The contrast in satisfaction between "user failure" (T-11) and "biologic failure" (T-9) underlines the difference in motivation.

Further investigation of the physiology of the pituitary-ovarian hormonal axis in relation to the cervical mucus will no doubt lead to much more refinement of the method, but the real key appears to be in the choices people make regarding their fertility as they understand it. Reproduction is a natural function of coital activity. For those who understand the likelihood of conception, the method works—even though the number of observations is limited. The comparison of the satisfaction levels discussed earlier in this paper corroborates the above statement. As is true for all methods of fertility control, as couples are followed a variety of outcomes appear. Our series reflects this. The terminology reflects a very strong contraceptive bias and does not serve the purpose of this study well because the study was aimed at fertility awareness and the choice consequent upon such awareness. Deeper study of the motivations underlying choices would be very helpful.

It is hoped that the log-rank method of statistical analysis will establish the significance of the Billings Ovulation Method as the sample size increases. Studies in progress, such as those funded by the Division of Population Research of the National Institutes of Health[13] and the Task Force on Human Reproduction of the World Health Organization, will corroborate or contradict this pilot study.

Acknowledgments. Special thanks are due to Kathy Platt and Martin Sharp, and the Data Control Center of St. Francis Hospital, Wichita, Kan.

REFERENCES

1. Billings EL, Billings JJ, Brown JB, Burger HG: Symptoms and hormonal changes accompanying ovulation. Lancet 1:282, 1972

2. Klaus H, Woods RE, Castles MR, Zimny GH: Behavioral components influencing use effectiveness of family planning by prediction of ovulation. In Proceedings of the 4th International Congress of Psychosomatic Obstetrics and Gynecology, Edited by H Hirsch. Basel, E Karger, 1974, p 218

3. Flynn A, Lynch SS: Cervical mucus and identification of the fertile phase of the menstrual cycle. Br J Obstet Gynaecol 83:656, 1976

4. Tietze C, Lewit S: Statistical evaluation of contraceptive methods. Clin Obstet Gynecol 17:121, 1974

5. Azen SP, Roy S, Pike MC, Casagrande J: Some suggested improvements to current statistical methods of analyzing contraceptive efficacy. J Chronic Dis 29:649, 1976

6. Tietze C, Lewit S: Use-effectiveness of oral and intrauterine contraception. Fertil Steril 22:508, 1971

7. Rice FJ, Lanctot CA, Garcia-Devasa C: Cited in periodic abstinence. Population Rep. Ser I, June 1974, p 12

8. Rötzer J: Erweiterte Basaltemperaturmessung und Empfangnisregelung. Arch Gynaekol 206:195, 1968

9. Lane ME, Arceo R, Sobrero AJ: Successful use of the diaphragm and jelly by a young population: report of a clinical study. Fam Plann Perspect 8:81, 1976

10. Dunn HP: Natural family planning. NZ Med J 82:407, 1975

11. Gupta HD, Devi PK, Gupta I: A Three year study of the Copper T 200 intrauterine device. Contraception 14:165, 1976

12. Barrett JC, Marshall J: Risk of conceptions. Population Stud 23:455, 1969

13. Corfman PA: Validation of the effectiveness of natural family planning. Presented at the Eighth World Congress of Gynecology and Obstetrics, Mexico City, October 17–22, 1976

Appendix 6
The Ovulation Method and the Menopause

Dr. Evelyn L. Billings

The menopause by strict definition is the physiological cessation of the menstrual periods, occurring towards the age of fifty years. It is more appropriate to discuss the climacteric or "change of life", by which is meant the gradual decline in reproductive capacity extending over several years, of which the menopause is one indication. Fertility progressively diminishes for several years until, in the age group of forty-five to fifty years, there is evidence that only 1.3 women per thousand are able to become pregnant; after the age of fifty about 1 in 25 thousand. Apart from the male sperm count, fertility depends upon the occurrence of ovulation and upon the presence of a mucus which assists conception. The menstrual periods may continue for months or years after the woman is no longer capable of conceiving, and her infertility may be the result either of a cessation of ovulation or of a failure to secrete satisfactory mucus. We have seen the reappearance of a typical fertile mucus pattern with succeeding menstruation for a number of cycles, after amenorrhea for a year or more, in this pre-menopausal group.

The management consists first of all in teaching the woman to understand her own pattern of fertility by careful instruction in the mucus and by instilling confidence to follow the simple rules which will enable her and her husband to avoid pregnancy, if this is what they wish. Many of the women I am reporting in this study had never been informed previously of the Ovulation Method; it is helpful if the women have come to understand it when the occurrence of more or less regular fertile cycles makes it so easy to learn.

We studied a consecutive group of 98 women for an average of three to four years, forty of them being aged between thirty-eight and forty-five, the remainder being over forty-five years of age. Most of them were anxious, or very anxious about the possibility of further pregnancies. The anxiety was sometimes a reflection of ignorance about the menopause, in others the appearance of marked irregularity in the menstrual cycles had made them realise that they could not longer follow the Rhythm Method, on which they had previously depended. Seventeen had had a recent pregnancy after years of successful usage of the Rhythm Method or a combination of the Temperature and Rhythm Methods. Prolonged abstinence had then been accepted, but had gradually provoked considerable marital disharmony with resultant depression. The husband, who was now feeling rejected, had begun to demand intercourse and to behave unreasonably in various ways, while at the same time, there was aggravation of the emotional disturbance by problems of their teenage children. It has been estimated that most of the psychological disturbances which have come to be associated with the menopause, are of psychic origin and that not more than 10% have any basis in hormonal disturbances.

There was one feature of all these women that was uniform—that they were all determined to find a natural solution to their problems and rejected all those methods of artificial contraception which had been offered them; they exhibited a touching confidence in our ability to help them, which provided a great impetus to the study.

With daily estimations of the urinary levels of oestrogens and progestogens we investigated the relationships of the various types of mucus observed to the hormonal pattern. The results showed quite clearly that the occurrence of ovulation is not itself sufficient to indicate fertility. There were many cycles observed in which the hormonal levels (and the basal body temperature record) showed a typical ovulatory pattern and yet the cervical mucus lacked the characteristics of fertility; in some of these cases intercourse had occurred at or just before the time of ovulation without conception as a result. The descriptions of the mucus varied although such expressions as "different", "dry", "crusty", "insignificant", "none at all", were commonly used. On a number of occasions the woman would notice the return of clear, lubricative mucus with Spinnbarkeit after many months of irregular "insignificant mucus" and erratic menstruation; she was then able to predict accurately the next menstrual period. Eight of the women in the over-forty-five group had levels of oestrogens between 100 and 214 micrograms, in 24 hours, and yet reported an "insignificant" mucus; certainly the development of a satisfactory mucus cannot be related in a linear fashion to the total oestrogen level.

THE HISTORY

At the first interview an estimate was made of the likely state of fertility on the basis of the woman's age, the number of children and miscarriages, the age of the youngest child, the method of avoiding pregnancy used since the last pregnancy and whether she had taken the contraceptive pill, as the tendency of this medication to produce prolonged sterility is especially evident at this age. The time of onset of irregularity of the menses and the cycle variation were also recorded in detail regarding the menstrual flow, such as alteration in length or volume, the presence of clots, etc. It is common for the menstrual periods to become short and scanty, or there may be prolonged spotting. In either cases there may be a considerable increase in the bleeding, even flooding. There may be bleeding between the periods and bleeding in close proximity to ovulation, even though such bleeding has not been observed earlier in life.

The breast tension which normally occurs during the post-ovulatory phase of the cycle may not disappear altogether; in some cases the absence of a fertile mucus pattern in addition suggests that this is an indication of the cycle being anovular. In other cases breast tension and soreness may be extremely severe, beginning before ovulation and continuing for a few weeks, even up to the time of the next period.

The "hot flush", by which is meant not merely an intolerance of a hot stuffy atmosphere, but a sudden feeling of heat in the upper limbs, the head and neck, for several seconds with rapid offset, is an indication of infertility and is accompanied by a low oestrogen level. The hot flushes may occur 20 to 30 times in the day, may wake the woman at night and may disappear for weeks or months only to return later. It used to be thought that hot flushes were a reliable indication of the end of the reproductive period of life but there is a lesson to be learned from the only woman in this series who became pregnant; she had observed hot flushes for some months with indication from the mucus pattern of infertility in her cycles but thereafter developed a typical fertile mucus pattern, ignored the rules for the avoidance of pregnancy and became pregnant. She had realised that she was very likely to be pregnant as a result of this act of intercourse, and correctly predicted that she would miss the menstrual period which would otherwise have followed this ovulation.

Other clinical features include weight gain, particularly loss of the waistline or "return to the neuter shape", as some writers have unattractively described it. Mood changes are common with unreasonable irritability and depression, sometimes severe depression, particularly associated with long heavy periods. One notices the association between "dry days", the hot flushes and very low oestrogen levels, indicating certain infertility at that time.

THE MANAGEMENT

Regular supervision, the woman being seen every week or so, is necessary at first, so that the details of any mucus which is observed can be discussed; the teacher soon discerns whether the woman can be depended upon to recognise any indications of fertility in the mucus, and gradually more and more days become available for intercourse without fear of pregnancy; domestic harmony is restored and confidence in the Method continues to develop.

Medical assessment is important, unusual bleeding or discharge being an indication for consultation. The hormonal patterns have often enabled the irregular bleeding to be explained, for example, as an oestrogen-withdrawal effect. We have not used synthetic oestrogen therapy for the hot flushes because it is a rather ineffective measure, because the oestrogens may themselves cause bleeding and because they may produce a secretion of mucus which creates confusion for the woman beginning to learn the Ovulation Method (though not when she is experienced). The practice of prescribing the contraceptive pill in order to restore more or less regular bleeding in order to alleviate anxiety is rejected altogether. Simple treatment for anaemia may be indicated but otherwise observation with resultant understanding is the recommended procedure; in this way much anxiety and unnecessary treatment can be avoided.

The precise details of the mucus symptom is carefully described (Billings 1973, Billings et alii, 1974) and, as usual, the woman and her husband are asked to accept a month's abstinence from all intimate sexual contact. A careful record of the physiological events of the day are made each evening, the woman using her own vocabulary to describe her observations. It is important to explain to the inexperienced woman that the normal fertile pattern of earlier years may have disappeared permanently, but that this does not prevent the successful application of the Ovulation Method.

The regular supervision and encouragement provided by the teacher are of inestimable value to the woman and her husband. In our initial instruction we are careful to inform the husbands of the significance of the menopause and the various problems which may be associated with it. It is helpful to promote some discussion between the men themselves, the leader being a husband who has experienced the successful application of the Ovulation Method for some considerable time.

RESULTS

In this particular series of 98 women, followed for an average of three to four years, the high level of motivation to avoid pregnancy was impressive. As is our constant practice, it was made absolutely clear to the women and their husbands that it was their personal prerogative to depart from the use of the Method at any time they wished. No request was made that any intention to become pregnant should be announced in advance; such a demand would immediately eliminate many people so that the study would no longer be comprehensive. Only one woman was lost to the series, and in her case this occurred because excessive irregular bleeding was unable to be controlled by medical treatment and was, therefore, treated by hysterectomy.

As previously described, we define a *Biological* or *Method-Failure* as a pregnancy which occurs when so far as can be ascertained, the couple has understood the instructions and carried them out faithfully. A *User-Failure* is defined as an error on the part of the couple which the teacher can ascertain and explain to their satisfaction. (Weissmann et alii, 1972.) There were no method-failures and no user-failures. Only one woman became pregnant, and this pregnancy was the result of putting to the test the observed and recognised indication provided by the cervical mucus symptom, that the day used for intercourse was a day of probable fertility.

This "menopausal" study is one illustration of the superiority of the Ovulation Method over the Rhythm Method, the Temperature Method, and the Temperature and Rhythm Methods combined. There is a statement by Tietze (1970) regarding the effectiveness of the Temperature Method, in which he, unfortunately, uses the title Temperature-Rhythm, when he really means the Temperature Method alone, and not Temperature-Rhythm combined. He says, "Temperature-Rhythm, i.e., the determination of ovulation by the basal body temperature and the restriction of coitus to the post-ovulatory phase of the cycle, also falls into the most highly effective group contraceptive method". He then goes on to say, "Its practice requires that all temperature curves be correctly recorded and interpreted, and that coitus be entirely avoided not only prior to ovulation but also in the post-ovulatory phase, if the curve is equivocal". There need be little wonder, therefore, that most statistical reports of the Temperature Method refer almost exclusively to women with more or less regular and fertile cycles, avoiding those with very long and highly irregular cycles, women who are breast-feeding, women who are approaching the menopause, and not always making it clear that all sexual contact had to be avoided in those cycles in which a definite biphasic temperature pattern was not obtained. All that, of course, was the position in May 1970, but now in August 1973 a different situation exists; the Ovulation Method provides warning of the approach of fertility, and those situations in which the thermometer is of little use or of no use at all, have found a solution.

Appendix 7
A Trial of the Ovulation Method of Family Planning in Tonga

Sister M. Cosmas Weissmann
Catholic missionary order of Marist nuns, Tonga

Leopino Foliaki
General Hospital, Tonga

Evelyn L. Billings
John J. Billings
*Family Planning Clinic, St. Vincent's Hospital,
Melbourne, Australia*

SUMMARY

In the ovulation method the woman defines the fertile and infertile days of her menstrual cycle by interpreting the cervical-mucus pattern. Clinical studies have shown that in all women the occurrence of fertility is accompanied by a characteristic mucous secretion, which allows the woman to recognise the days when conception is likely. This information provides a "natural" method of family planning, and a trial of its potential value was undertaken in a Pacific Island community. The method proved to be both acceptable and successful. Altogether 282 women used the ovulation method for a total of 2503 months, with one case of method failure and two cases of user failure.

INTRODUCTION

The ovulation method[1] was developed to overcome the weaknesses of the rhythm method and the temperature method. The ovulation method is based on the known association in animals and humans of a characteristic type of cervical mucus, and usually an actual mucous discharge, at about the time of ovulation; it involves the instruction of women in the accurate interpretation of a symptom with which they are already quite familiar. The ability of women to recognise this symptom has already been assessed.[2] We found that even unintelligent and uneducated women were able to use the method successfully, either to avoid or to achieve pregnancy.

Doubts have been expressed about the probable success of a method of family planning which demands periodic abstinence in a "primitive" community. An opportunity to undertake a trial of the method in Tonga presented itself in 1970 when M. C. W. visited Melbourne, after many years' experience as a teacher and a nurse in Tonga, during which time she had become fluent in the native tongue.

Tonga seemed to be a suitable area for clinical trial of the ovulation method. The people are Polynesian, gentle, friendly, and easy-going in their outlook. Very few women are aware of the length of their menstrual cycles. The practice of coitus interruptus is common, there is a general lack of motivation to limit the family's size despite poverty, and a consequent tendency to resist the application of methods involving continuing supervision and personal effort, whatever claims for success are made in their promotion.

The total population of the Tongan Kingdom is about 90,000 people, scattered over a total of 150 islands which cover an area of 250 square miles. The economy is wholly dependent upon agricultural products, and diet contains a large amount of carbohydrate. Only one person in five is gainfully employed, but most people have enough to eat. Primary-school education is compulsory and some medical services are free. European civilisation has made some impact on the inhabitants, but the majority are still rather unsophisticated, generally having difficulty in sustaining attempts at material advancement.

Instruction in family planning involved extensive travel around the islands by car, bicycle, and boat. In many areas only occasional visits were possible, separated by intervals of months. This necessitated taking up residence in various localities until a proper understanding of the method had been reached. The acceptance of the method was a voluntary decision made by both husband and wife. They were free to learn the method, to use it at once or later if they wished, and they were promised assistance whenever it was required, on the understanding that they would always be free to abandon the method and to return to it again.

The usual technique was to gather the women and their husbands together on a Sunday evening and to outline the method. The need for the couple's mutual cooperation in avoiding sexual contact when the mucus indicated possible fertility was emphasised. It has proved a considerable advantage to instruct the men, not only for the individual couple, but also because the men help to spread the information to other couples in their villages. People of "advanced cultures" have suggested that men living in more primitive communities will not tolerate sexual restraint. Our experience has shown this to be false, both by the ready acceptance of the husbands of a period of continence and by the abandonment of the habit of coitus interruptus in the vast majority instructed. There was strong male cooperation despite the relaxed life of the island, which would not be regarded as conducive to sexual restraint. The strong motivation of women who used the method successfully was partly the result of their husbands' insistence that they cooperate with the teacher.

On the following morning the women attended for more detailed instruction, when there was free discussion of the details of the mucus symptom. Some general instruction on anatomy and physiology was provided, with an explanation of ovulation and its occurrence approximately two weeks before the next menstrual period. It was explained that, unlike the rhythm method, the ovulation method does not require regular menstrual cycles, nor the keeping of a calendar. The phases of the menstrual cycle were outlined—the menstrual period, the "dry days", and the "mucus days". The change in the physical characteristics of the mucus close to ovulation was described in detail, the appearance of clear or stretchy or slippery mucus being the reliable indication of fertility. Emphasis was placed on both the appearance of the mucus and the lubricative sensation produced by this "fertile" mucus—the "peak" symptom which the women find easy to recognise. It was also explained that during long cycles, during breast-feeding, &c., "patches of mucus", that is, a succession of days on which mucus may be observed, occur intermittently before the typical pattern of a fertile ovulation, and that until the woman is experienced in the method sexual contact must be avoided whenever mucus is present. The scanty-mucus pattern of infertile cycles was also explained, and the need to distinguish the loss of seminal fluid after intercourse from the mucus symptom, an ability which is quickly attained.

A simple method of recording this information by the use of red, green, and white stamps was developed in Central America, and this was of great practical value. This record keeping, especially during the first few cycles after instruction, has the advantage of training the women to understand the symptom and of providing the teacher with a record of the progress of the instruction. The women also helped one another by comparing and discussing individual records. In each locality the women were seen at least weekly, or more frequently if necessary, so that additional instruction could be given and confidence in the method gained.

INITIAL RESPONSE

In the first few months, when the teaching method was being developed, some women expressed difficulty in understanding the mucus symptom, a few complained of persistent vaginal discharges, and there were some reports of pregnancies which were interpreted as failures of the method until the areas involved were revisited and the circumstances in which these pregnancies had occurred determined. There was resistance in some cases to efforts to persuade the husband and wife to abandon the coitus interruptus which initially was practised by about 85% in those receiving instruction. A suggestion to use the thermometer was rejected because practical experience had shown that a large-scale use of the temperature method was impossible, both because of the expense involved and more especially because the method necessitates constant supervision. In addition, it was recognised that the temperature method is inferior to the ovulation method because it defines only days of infertility after ovulation, and even in that is less precise than the ovulation method. Tonga has its own special problem, in that prolonged breast-feeding is common and basal-temperature measurement cannot give warning of the resumption of ovulation. The temperature method also does not give information on infertility during anovular cycles.

It was essential to warn the husband and wife that coitus interruptus during the fertile phase of the cycle cannot be expected reliably to prevent pregnancy. Therefore, only those couples who were prepared to abandon the practice were accepted into the survey, there being no intention of allowing either the successful prevention of pregnancy by coitus interruptus to be recorded as a success for the ovulation method or a failure of coitus interruptus to be recorded as a failure of the ovulation method. Additionally, acts of sexual intercourse, including coitus interruptus, during the presence of the cervical mucus make the assessment of the symptom more difficult and therefore delay or prevent the correct interpretation of the symptom. The great majority of couples soon agreed to discontinue coitus interruptus, with a predictable increase in the physical and emotional satisfaction they derived from the act of intercourse.

Pathological vaginal discharges were seldom a problem. They can usually be treated successfully and in any event do not prevent the woman from recognising the time of fertility by the change produced in the pathological discharge by the characteristic mucus. In those women with a protracted mucus symptom additional detailed instruction was given to increase the freedom for intercourse by defining "relatively safe days" when "infertile" mucus was present and by avoiding sexual contact on any days when clear or stretchy or slippery mucus was observed; these individual problems lessened with increasing experience on the part of the woman herself and of the teacher.

THE GROUP STUDIED

We report 395 women who were instructed after the start of the project in July, 1970; the results were assessed in February, 1972.

There was a good response to the instruction. 331 couples opted for the ovulation method. Most women found the mucus symptom immediately recognisable, and were pleased by the simplicity of the method. Many reacted favourably because they preferred a "natural" method, some because of the psychological advantage of a solution which is obtained by mutual cooperation, and some because of the attitude of the teacher, which never contained any element of coercion. The possibility of the information being employed to help those women whose marriages had been infertile created additional interest, and of the total there were 18 women who were anxious to become pregnant. 46 couples elected to use another method to avoid pregnancy, including one case in which the woman discovered that she had been sterilised at the time of a previous caesarean operation. The preference expressed by these couples was as follows:

METHOD	NUMBER
Coitus interruptus	27
I.U.C.D.	5
Contraception (unspecified)	9
Condom	2
Contraceptive medication	1
Rhythm method	1
Sterilisation (involuntary)	1

In the assessment of the results care was taken to make allowance for other influences which could have contributed to success. Coitus interruptus has already been mentioned. The ancient custom of a period of abstinence after childbirth has now fallen into disuse, intercourse being resumed after childbirth within an average of 5 to 6 weeks, this time being unaffected by a decision to suckle the child or not.

Many women were instructed during pregnancy or immediatley after childbirth. In all cases the time on the method was not measured until at least six weeks after the confinement. If the mother was feeding the child herself the time was calculated from the date on which solid food was introduced into the weaning diet, however long after the confinement this proved to be. It is a matter of experience that a number of the Tongan women do become pregnant again whilst fully breast-feeding their infants, but as breast-feeding does reduce fertility ten women were eliminated from the total on this account; they are nevertheless established on the method, and none has become pregnant. 14 women were eliminated from the assessment because it was judged that they were close to the menopause; they were forty-three years of age or older, had irregular menstrual cycles and a scanty mucus symptom; they too have followed the method by avoiding intimate sexual contact on days when mucus has been observed, and none has become pregnant. There were retained in the series 17 women aged 41 to 45 years in whom there was no clinical evidence of approaching menopause; all the remaining women were younger. There were 2 women who were discovered to have been already pregnant at the initial interview. One woman has been lost to follow-up. 18 couples decided that they would postpone use of the method until they had had more children. 4 couples were eliminated because of separation, 1 husband having died, 2 having travelled overseas to seek employment, and 1 woman having required protracted confinement in hospital for mental illness; even when this woman was allowed home she was obviously unwell, and intercourse occurred infrequently (see table I).

TABLE 1.   Total cases for analysis of results

—	NO.
Couples learning method to avoid pregnancy when desired	331
Anxious for more children at present	18
No recent information	1
Separated	4
Pregnant at initial interview	2
Still fully breast-feeding	10
Menopausal (age, irregular cycles, scanty mucus)	14
Total remaining	282

We encourage couples learning the method to refrain from sexual contact during the first cycle after instruction, so that the woman's understanding of the mucus symptom is not hindered by the effects of sexual intercourse. This recommendation was not insisted upon and not followed by all couples. However, to avoid loading the statistics in favour of success by the elimination of "high-risk cases", the time has been counted from the start of instruction and all have been included. There were two cases of the women having been uncertain of the correct application of the method; in both these cases the error was understood after further explanation.

There were 28 couples who, after following the method carefully for several months, elected to abandon it because they were anxious to have more children. The prompt occurrence of pregnancy when intercourse occurs on a day of clear, stretchy or slippery "fertile mucus" increases the confidence that couples have already developed in the reliability of the method. All of these couples intend to use the method again after confinement, and some are already doing so.

There were 50 women who "took a chance" by having intercourse on a day when the presence of the mucus had been recognised, and who therefore had no difficulty in realising why pregnancy had occurred. All of these women except one, who finds the observation of the mucus symptom and the period of abstinence troublesome, intend to use the method again in the future and many are already doing so. There is only one woman who believes that she did not have any sexual contact on a day in which the mucus warned her of possible fertility; she too, however, although apparently a "method-failure", is now using the method again, and successfully (see table II).

TABLE 2.   Analysis of 81 Pregnancies

—	NO.
Couples using method	282
Subsequently pregnant	81
Abandoned method, desiring more children	28
Ignored indication of possible fertility	50
Used mucus day, thought infertile	2
Considers no days of possible fertility used	1
Average age (yr.) of women who deliberately or carelessly abandoned the method	33·2
Average number of children	4·8
Average age (yr.) of women still successfully applying the method	33·7
Average number of children	6·8

RESULTS

The pregnancies which occurred, other than by design or by the conscious neglect of the instructions, were classified in one of two ways:

A biological or method-failure was recorded when, so far as could be ascertained, the couple had understood and carried out the instructions faithfully.

A user failure was recorded when there was an error on the part of the couple which the teacher could ascertain and explain to them to their satisfaction.

Altogether in this series a total of 282 women used the ovulation method for a total of 2503 months. There were two cases of user failure and one case of method failure.

Of the 18 women who were anxious to conceive, 7 subsequently became pregnant after careful attention to the mucus symptom and concentrating acts of intercourse in that part of the cycle when the peak symptom was in evidence. Previous investigation has shown that this peak-symptom day when the mucus is clearer than at other times, when it is stringy and produces a definite lubricative sensation, is on the average 0·9 days before ovulation.[2] Knowing that it is necessary for the spermatozoa to be in the female genital tract for some hours in order for them to become capable of fertilising the ovum, the day of the peak symptom is taken as the day of maximum fertility.

One of the women classified as a user failure had a long cycle in which mucus was observed on a succession of days. She had then incorrectly concluded that she had passed ovulation and had intercourse later in the cycle, on a day when copious amounts of clear slippery mucus were present. Explicit instruction is now given regarding the possibility of recurrent days of mucus in long cycles, in order for this mistake to be avoided, with emphasis on the avoidance of sexual contact when a fertile type of mucus is observed.

The second woman classified as a user failure had reported some confusion about the instructions, and uncertainty regarding the definition of fertile and infertile days. This pregnancy miscarried in July, 1971, after which she recommenced the use of the ovulation method; when last seen in March, 1972, she had become quite confident, and was using the method successfully.

The woman who was classified as a "method-failure", because she was unaware of having used a day when any mucus was present, received her initial instruction immediately after a confinement, before ovulation and menstruation had recommenced. The child which was conceived after instruction was born in September, 1971, and since then the woman has been using the ovulation method successfully.

DISCUSSION

There is in Tonga a Government-sponsored birth-control programme which provides contraceptive medication, intrauterine devices, &c., free. The interest of the people in the natural method is therefore in spite of these other provisions. Approximately 75% of the women who came for instruction were Catholics.

Establishment on the method is accompanied by feelings of relief and freedom. Many women quickly determine to pass on the information about the method to other women, and in particular to instruct their daughters so that they, too, can space their families. It is essential that the method be taught by a woman who is devoted to the success of a natural method and that the teaching be kept quite separate from that of any other method of family planning. It is not essential that the teacher should have had medical training; most women learn to become competent teachers after charting and studying their own cycles for a few months. An essential point which is emphasised in the instruction is that the women study carefully the sensation produced by the presence of the mucus, as well as noting its appearance.

It assists understanding of the method when women are reminded that they may have infertile cycles from time to time, in which little mucus is evident, and that this does not prevent the successful application of the method. Many "infertile" women notice that the typical mucus occurs in very few cycles, or not at all; instruction will acquaint these women of their greatest chance of achieving pregnancy, and will provide the information in time for it to be applied.

In the early months of this project a number of difficulties had to be overcome and the teaching programme organised. There were a number of women who found the interpretation of the mucus symptom difficult at first, and there were cases where the husband and wife found the periodic abstinence a problem. As we have observed in other circumstances, the abstinence became less of a problem when confidence in the method was established and the practice of coitus interruptus eliminated.

This investigation has demonstrated that the ovulation method is capable of successful application in a Pacific-Island community. The extraordinarily high success-rate is to be attributed to several factors:

(1) The teacher was a woman. She was an experienced teacher as well as a trained nurse, and most of the women instructed had been taught by her in their school days, so that she knew something of their character, ability, and dispostions.

(2) The teacher lived with the people during the learning period, so that she could provide individual advice and attention.

(3) The couples were living far from the pressures of modern civilisation. Possibly they have a greater awareness of physiological changes in the body than people in more sophisticated communities. The women were aware of the presence of the mucus and were able to recognise the peak symptom, contrary to the expectation of some people without experience of enlightened teaching of the method.

(4) Strong motivation on the part of the women came in many cases from the influence of their husbands, who insisted that their wives cooperate with the teacher.

It may be more difficult to achieve a similar degree of success in all communities, especially in those where sexual permissiveness is fashionable. Our experience in Tonga has shown that the method works. The explanation for failures is to be found in inadequate teaching or in a lack of cooperation and motivation by the persons concerned.

It has been most gratifying that those couples who "broke the rule" have, if anything, greater confidence in the method as a result, and have willingly returned to its use subsequently.

His Lordship, John H. Rodgers, Bishop of Tonga, met the expenses of this project, and we thank him for his consistent encouragement.

Requests for reprints should be addressed to J. J. B., St. Vincent's Hospital, Victoria Parade, Melbourne 3065, Australia.

REFERENCES

1. Billings, J. J. The Ovulation Method. Melbourne, 1972.
2. Billings, E. L., Billings, J. J., Brown, J. B., Burger, H. G. Lancet, 1972, i, 282.

Appendix 8
Preliminary Report of Use-Effectiveness of Ovulation Method in Korea

Kyu Sang Cho, M.D.
Korea Happy Family Movement Association

For a retrospective study of the presurvey data analysis and use-effectiveness from April 1, 1975 to Nov., 30, 1975, we have dealt with a total of 1,383 women, (urban areas 465, rural areas 918).

The results of preliminary survey were as follows:

1. Number of women observed: 1,383
   Number of menstrual cycles: 11,064
   Failure rate: 13.56 (on the basis of pregnancies per 100 women-years on Pearl Formula)
2. Among 465 women in urban areas, the failure rate was 10.32, which signified unplanned pregnancies of 32 women.
   27 of the 32 women were pregnant due to the users' own failure and the remaining 5 due to the failure of the method.
   Therefore, the failure of the method accounted for 1.41.
3. Among 918 rural women, the failure rate was 15.19 signifying unplanned pregnancies in 93 women.

The cause of the failure in 81 of the 93 women was attributable to the users' own mistake and that in the remaining 12 to the default of the method.
Therefore, the failure attributable to the method accounted for 1.96.

Extended Use-Effectiveness of Cervical Mucus Method, Calculated on the Basis of Pregnancies per 100 Woman-Years (Pearl Formula)

CERVICAL MUCUS METHOD	NO. OF WOMEN	NO. OF MENSTRUAL CYCLES	NO. OF UNPLANNED PREGNANCIES	FAILURE RATE (PREGNANCIES/ 100 WOMAN-YEARS)
Author, 1975	1,383	11,064	125	13.56
Weissmann, Foliaki, Billings & Billings, Tonga, 1972	282	2,503	3	1.4
Marshall, 1972 (analysis of Weissmann data in retrospect)	282	2,503	53	25.4

Extended Use-Effectiveness of Cervical Mucus Method in Different Areas Calculated on the Basis of Pregnancies per 100 Woman-Years (Pearl Formula) 1975

	NO. OF WOMEN	NO. OF PLANNED PREGNANCIES	NO. OF ACCIDENTAL PREGNANCIES	USER'S FAILURE RATE	METHOD'S FAILURE RATE	FAILURE RATE
Urban	465	29	32	8.71 (27)	1.61 (5)	10.32
Rural	918	81	93	13.24 (81)	1.96 (12)	15.19

( ): No. of Pregnancies

Methods of Contraception Before Use of Ovulation Method (urban areas)

METHOD	NO.	%
Oral pill	112	24.08
Condom	81	17.42
Loop	45	9.68
Rhythm method	56	12.04
Extravaginal ejaculation	23	4.95
Cervical mucus method	10	2.15
Subtotal	327	70.32
No Use	138	29.68
Total	465	100

Appendix 9
The Use Effectiveness of the Ovulation Method in India

M. M. Mascarenhas
A. Lobo
A. S. Ramesh et al*

ABSTRACT

This study of the Ovulation Method by CREST Centre for Research, Education, Service and Training for Family Life Promotion, 21, Museum Road, Bangalore-560025, evaluated 3530 acceptors from January 1975 through December 1977. This evaluation was done through determining the aggregate and average women months of use, the net cumulative continuation rates, Pearls' Pregnancy rates and Life Table Pregnancy Rates.

The Life Table Analysis showed that this method has greater acceptability and higher use effectiveness as compared to other spacing methods.

INTRODUCTION

Natural Family planning by the Symptothermic and Ovulation Method was introduced into general usage in India from 1966 onwards.[1] This paper on the Ovulation Method is a collaborative study of several centres from various states of India.[2]

The Ovulation Method (OM) Billings is a fertility-awareness method whereby a woman observes, records and interprets her genital sensations during her menstrual cycle.

The Centre for Research, Education, Service and Training for Family Life Promotion (CREST) is presently also engaged in a Research Study of the Ovulation Method (WHO Multicentre Trial and the Karnataka Study, both directed by CREST Bangalore).

This paper is the first study of the Ovulation Method using accepted rules and methodology in India. It was the only method used by the study population.

*Dr. Marie Mignon Mascarenhas,, FRIPHH., MBBS., MFCM., DPH. (Lond.) is the Director of CREST (Centre for Research, Education, Service and Training for Family Life Promotion) of the Family Welfare Centre, Bangalore and Principal Investigator for India in the Clinical Multicentre Trial of the WHO.
* Dr. Aloma Lobo, M.B.B.S., Assistant Director of Crest, and the Principal Teacher WHO Trial.
* Mr. A. S. Ramesh, M.Sc., is the Associate Research and Evaluation Officer of the Community Health and Family Planning Project of the Christian Medical Association of India.
ET AL—The Teacher, doctors, nurses of all the Centres participating in the Study.

The Programme Evaluation of 3,530 Acceptors over a period of 36 months from January 1975 through December 1977, with December 1977 as the cut off point.

Materials & Methods

The Centres partcipating were located in several States[2] of India thus giving a varied picture of all cultures and socio-economic classes. Commonly adopted methods of record keeping, data collection and terminology were used viz, a Chart (plain ruled paper) and a red and blue pencil at a total cost of 40p. or 12 cents US., for 1 year. Approx 50% of the clients were recruited by satisfied users. All the investigators were trained by CREST.

CREST has 18 Sub-centres in and around Bangalore. Four hospitals have NFP Clinics, of which St. Martha's Hospital was used as the Chief referral centre, (for Gynaecological or other investigations) whenever necessary.

The Ovulation Method

Is based on self recognition by the women of her fertile and infertile period by the subjective sensation of wetness in her genital areas. It has been described first by Billings[3]−The crypts of the cervix secret E (oestrogenic) type mucus[4] in response to Oestrogenic stimulation which is also responsible for ovulation (release of ovum or egg from the ovary). A "trigger-like" mechanism goes into action when the oestrogen level reaches a peak and a simultaneous response is evoked[5] from the Ovary and cervical crypts as this peak approaches. Thus ovulation and fertile mucus secretion occur simultaneously. Ovulation is hypothesized to occur from 9 hours before to 48 hours after the peak of wetness, hence all of the mucus days preceeding the "peak symptom" plus 72 hours following are the presumed fertile days of the couple.[6] Specifically the cervical mucus secretion gives a typical sensation which indicates the fertile days, and warns her of impending ovulation.

She is also trained to observe mucus at the vulva. In view of the fact that neither toilet paper nor underwear is used by the majority of our sari-clad women, precedence is given to sensation. Women with leucorrhoea or cervicitis were treated and could follow the method satisfactorily.

The woman is asked to keep a daily record of sensation and/or discharge with a red and blue pencil on a chart. The supervising teacher keeps a duplicate chart. Red indicates menstruation or spotting. Blue, the dry days. A circle with a dot within indicates the wet days. Peak by a cross on a wet day recognized as peak.

Illiterate women find this recording easy. The record is made at night, or late evening. This visual impression is important for the husband who at a glance knows the fertile status of his wife.

A USER is a woman currently utilizing the method within the context of exposure to sexual intercourse.

A couple abstains from sexual intercourse during the fertile phase of the menstrual cycle. Non genital communications or expressions are encouraged during the period of abstinence so that marital happiness can be increased and even stabilised by focusing on verbal communication.

Criteria for Admission into Study

To be admitted into the study a woman must have been below 44 years of age with a history of regular spontaneous menstrual cycles at intervals of 23–35 days. If neither postpartum nor post-lactation, she should have had two cycles prior to admission to the study. Subjects should have ceased breastfeeding and must have had at least one menstrual period prior to admission.

She must be informed and willing to maintain the required records herself. All couples must be cohabitating. Volunteer couples must agree not to use any other method of fertility regulation during the study period and must be willing in principle to use this technique for fertility regulation during a period of 16 cycles.

RESULTS

Programme Evaluation Material for the Study

The evaluation of programe is carried out through:

  i. Aggregate and average women months of use
 ii. Net cumulative continuation rates and
iii. Pearls' Pregnancy rates, Life Table Pregnancy rates

For computation of these rates complete follow up data related to 3,530 acceptors over a period of 36 months from January 1975 through December 1977, with December 1977 as the cut off point, have been used.

Of these 3,530 women 499 (12.7%) had discontinued the method at various points of time. The aggregate women months of use was found to be 39,967 yielding an average of 11.3 months which is observed fairly high compared to any other method of spacing like the oral pills and IUD. (Simha et al 1972; Sadashivah et al 1973, 1974).[7]

Net Cumulative Continuation Rates:

Computed on the basis of modified life table technique are shown in Appendix A. At the end of the 6th month, continuation rate was 88.5% and as at cut off point there still were 80% continuing in the programme. The net cumulative continuation rates noticed in this study was comparatively higher than the rates in other studies.[8] (Sadashivaiah et all 1974; Murthy et all 1967; Simha et all 1972; Sadashivaiah et al 1974; Leela Mehra et al 1970).

Of the 449 discontinued cases 174 (38.8%) had failed to use the method properly, thus causing pregnancy. There were two cases of "Method failure", that had resulted in pregnancy. Both of these method failures occurred within four months use of the method. Thus, there were 176 pregnancies among the acceptors of this method during the study period. The Pearls' pregnancy rate was found to be 5.3 for all pregnancies. The Life Table pregnancy rate was found to be 5.7 at the end of one year. The Pearls' rate and the life table were almost the same in this study. The evaluation indicates that this method has greater acceptability and higher use effectiveness as compared to other spacing methods.[9]

TABLE I   Net cumulative continuation rates for the acceptors of NFP (Mucus) Method.

TABLE II Life Table Pregnancy rates for the NFP acceptors

APPENDIX A

TABLE 1.   Net Cumulative Continuation Rates for the Acceptors of NFP (Mucus) Method

ORDINAL MONTH	NET CUMULATIVE CONTINUATION RATES
3	91.3
6	88.5
9	87.5
12	87.1
18	86.3
24	85.5
30	82.3
36	80.2

TABLE 2.   Life Table Pregnancy Rates for the NFP Acceptors.

ORDINAL MONTHS	PREGNANCY RATES
3	2.7
6	4.6
9	5.3
12	5.7
15	6.0
18	6.6

$$\text{Pearl's Pregnancy rate} = \frac{176}{39.967} \times 1200$$

$$\text{(for all pregnancies)} = 5.3$$

$$\text{Life Table Pregnancy Rate} = 5.7 \quad \text{at the end of 12 months.}$$

DISCUSSION

"Family Planning literature abounds with examples of misguided attempts to change people's customs and traditions. It is easier, cheaper and more effective to supply what people will accept".[10]

A Study of 3,530 acceptors using the Ovulation Method (Billings) over a 36 month period is reported in the preceeding pages.

The Life Table Analysis showed that this method has greater acceptability and higher use effectiveness as compared to other spacing methods.

Counselling for marital harmony is an integral part of the teaching of this method. Latz and Reiner had concluded in their study that methods based on periodic abstinence are practical and reliable.[11] This was also confirmed more recently by Klaus et al.[12]

It may be concluded that the Ovulation Method should find wide acceptance in India.

ACKNOWLEDGMENT

The Authors express their indebtedness to the couples and teachers who participated so wholeheartedly in this Study.

Also to Dr. (Mrs) H. M. Sharma, Executive Director CMA1 Community Health & Family Planning Project for her constructive criticism and suggestions.

To our secretary Anne Galway for typing the manuscript, and Margaret Raj for scrutinising the date.

REFERENCES

1. Mascarenhas, M. M. 1975, "N.F.P. in India" Bangalore Family Welfare Centre
2. Andhara Pradesh, Karnataka, Kerala, West Bengal and Tamil Nadu.
3. Billings, J. J. 1964, The Ovulation Method, Melbourne Advocate Press.
4. W. H. O. Colloquim, 1973, Cervical Mucus in Human Reproduction, Geneva, W. H. O.
5. Burger, H. G., 1977 "The Process of Ovulation in Humans" Cali, Colombia, Proceedings International Conference.
6. Klaus H. et all: Billings Ovulation Method, April 1977. Second Year Study Bulletin Indian Federation of Medical Guilds.
7. (i) Mehra L., Mohapatra P. S., Sharma B. B. L., "A Report of the Oral Pill Pilot Project Clinics in India", CFPI technical paper No. 9, September 1970, New Delhi.
   (ii) Murthy D. V. R., Mohapatra P. A., and Prabhakar A. K. "An Analysis of Data on IUCD cases" CFPI, New Delhi 1968
   (iii) Sadashivaiah, K. and Subba Rao, M S., "The Statistical evaluation of IUCD in selected Mission Hospitals"–A two year follow-up". Journal of Bio-social Science London, May 1973
   (iv) Sadashivaiah, K., Ramesh A. S., Simha J. S., "A retrospective study of Oral acceptors in member Mission hospitals of the Southern Region". Journal of CMAI, October 1975. Also presented at the Seminar of Family Planning Research Studies held at Institute for Rural Health and Family Planning, Gandhigram, January 1976.
   (v) Simha, J. S., and Ramesh A. S., "Comparative Study of Oral Pill–Acceptors in the three member mission hospitals of Mysore State" The Journal of CMAI, October 1972.
8. Ibid 7
9. References for Pregnancy rates and Continuation rates.
   (i) Wan Fook Kee, Chen Ai Ju and Jessie Tan-Oral contraceptive Continuation rates in the Singapore National Program. Studies in Family Planning. Vol. 6, No. 1. January 1975 pp. 17–21.
   Pregnancy rates;
   at the end of 12 months–11.1 per cent
   at the end of 18 months–13.8 per cent

CONTINUATION RATES:	ORDINAL MONTHS	CONTN. RATE
	12	47.5
	18	39.9
	24	34.6
	36	28.9

   (ii) John E. Laing-Differentials in Contraceptive use effectiveness in the Phillippines. Studies in family Planning. Vol. 5, No. 10 October 1974. pp. 302–313.

Continuation Rates by Method. All Method continuation rates.

ORDINAL MONTH	PILL	IUD	RHYTHM	OTHERS
6	76.3	92.5	70.9	68.6
12	66.4	85.8	52.5	56.4
18	57.2	80.1	47.1	46.8
24	50.2	73.1	46.0	0

(iii) Miguel Pulido and Anthony R. Meashan—Two year results of a clinical study of the Tou—200 IUD—studies in Family Planning, Vol. 5, No. 7. U.S.A. July 1974 pp. 221–223.

ORDINAL MONTH	PREGNANCY RATE	CONTINUATION RATE
3	0.3	96.4
6	0.8	91.8
9	1.1	87.3
12	2.0	82.5
18	3.1	73.9
24	3.1	64.3

10. David H. P. R. "Acceptors and Acceptability" Populi Vol. 14 No. 41977 U.N.F.P.A. New York.
11. Latz, L. J. and Reiner E. C., "Failures in Natural Conception Control and their causes". Illinois Medical Journal 1937 Illinois.
12. Ibid 6.

Appendix 10
Study Confirms Values of Ovulation Method

SR. Leona Dolack, OSF, RN

Approximately 10 million women in the United States were reported in 1975 as using oral contraceptives for birth control.[1] While women continue to take the pill, much information and many studies are published about the hazards and side effects of these drugs in relationship to thromboembolism; gall bladder, liver, and heart diseases; hypertension; carcinogenic potentials; and possible fetal damage.

The reports of Inman and Vessey and Brickerstaff suggest a relationship between oral contraceptives and the occurrence of vascular embolization. Risk is greatest for women who take preparations containing a higher dose of estrogen.[2,3] Hellman's paper, based on the reports of many physicians around the country, holds that the safety of contraceptive pills is highly suspect.[4]

The association of breast cancer and the use of oral contraceptive drugs in both England and the United States is inconclusive.[5,6,7,8] Yet studies recommend caution and prolonged surveillance through pelvic and breast examinations of women of all ages using oral contraceptives. Studies with a significant number of women over a longer period of time will be necessary to obtain the true significance of the relationship between the use of oral contraceptives and carcinogenic disease because tumor development is associated with a long latency period.[9]

Liver disease associated with the use of oral contraceptives probably is related to the dosage of estrogen.[10] Reports from Great Britain and the United States describe hepatic adenomas in women taking oral contraceptives.[11,12] Editorials in *The Lancet* and the *British Medical Journal* state that no proven link exists between benign liver tumors and oral contraceptives. Women who have active or chronic liver disease, however, and those who have developed idiopathic jaundice of pregnancy are believed to increase their risk of tumors with the use of the pill.[13,14] Further research is needed to establish valid, conclusive evidence about the cause and effect relationship between liver disease and the contraceptive pills.

Studies reported by the Royal College of Practitioners and by a Boston drug surveillance program suggest an increased incidence of cholecystitis or cholelithiasis. The Royal College reports 68 cases per 100,000 users per year.[15] The Boston studies estimate 158 cases per

Sr. Leona is administrative assistant and director, Natural Family Planning Program, St. Vincent Hospital, Green Bay, WI.

100,000 users per year.[16] The British study indicates that the increased number of women with gall bladder disease coincides with increased progesterone content in the pill. The study reported that gallstones developed about four years after the pill was initiated.

The association of oral contraceptives and fetal damage has also been studied. These reports show a relationship between the use of oral contraceptives and fetal cardiac abnormalities, congenital limb-reduction defects, a higher incidence of twinning, and an increased number of first-trimester spontaneous abortions.[17,18,19,20,21,22] At present, it is not clear what in the contraceptive pill causes fetal damage.

The occurrence of hypertensive disease was found to be 1½ times greater in those using contraceptive pills as in never users, and the incidence rate for current users was six times that of individuals who never used a contraceptive pill.[23]

CONCERN LEADS TO INTEREST IN NATURAL METHODS

Rather than take a "wait and see" attitude, couples are seeking an alternative to chemical methods of family planning. Concern over reported side effects, health hazards, and inconclusive scientific results has increased interest in natural methods of family planning. And interest is growing in the new ovulation for Billings method or family planning.

Research leading to the discovery of the ovulation method dates to 1855, when Smith recognized the cyclic changes in the quantity and quality of cervical mucus.[24] It was not until 1933 that the relationship between these changes and the menstrual cycle was demonstrated. Sezuy and Vimeaux reported that the cervical discharge increased in volume and decreased in viscosity between the tenth and fifteenth day of a normal menstrual cycle.[25] Later, Sezuy and co-workers associated the increase in the volume of discharge first to the rise in urinary estrogen and then to the timing of ovulation.[26] Further studies in the 1940s confirmed that peak secretions coincided with ovulation.[27,28,29] Billings and colleagues determined ovulation by monitoring menstrual cycles in daily estimates of the total urinary output of estriol, estrone, estradiol, and pregnanediol. Along with these findings there were changes in the cervical mucus, from a cloudy, tacky mucus to a clear, slippery, stringy mucus and back to the cloudy, tacky type. The clear, slippery mucus corresponded with the peaking of estrogen in the cycle, indicating ovulation.[30]

A guide to periodic abstinence relying on changes in the cervical mucus was recommended by Billings in 1964.[31] The Billings method allows women to determine the fertile time in the menstrual cycle. It proposes that the mucus secretions that accompany ovulation offer a direct indication of oncoming ovulation and that, therefore, there is no need for a calendar or basal thermometer. As a result, sexual intercourse can take place during the pre- and postovulatory infertile days with relative assurance of infertility.[32]

The ovulation method, therefore, purports to offer an alternative and risk-free method of family planning that, if effective, can be utilized throughout a couple's reproductive lifetime. Since women learn to distinguish fertility by observing their mucus pattern, the method could be useful for all women—including those who had been on the pill, have just given birth, are premenopausal, or have irregular cycles. The method can be used successfully to prevent pregnancy or to achieve pregnancy. The purpose of the study described below was to evaluate the effectiveness as well as the satisfaction in using the ovulation method of family planning.

ST. VINCENT STUDY OF OVULATION METHOD

Methodology. In January 1975, St. Vincent Hospital, Green Bay, WI. developed a natural family planning program whereby trained couples taught the ovulation method.

After couples attend a class presentation of the ovulation method, each couple is counseled in private on a monthly basis until they are secure in using the method. Records containing pertinent data and information on all private counseling sessions are kept on each couple.

Under the auspices of St. Vincent Hospital, a study was conducted of all 435 couples who attended the Natural Family Planning Program in 1975. One year after each couple had gained confidence in using the ovulation method, a follow-up questionnaire was mailed to them to determine the effectiveness of the method as well as satisfaction in its use.*Nonrespondents were telephoned in order to complete the study. Three hundred seventy-one, or 82 percent, responded, and 82 were lost to the study, which was analyzed during spring and summer of 1977.

The women who became pregnant were asked to review their charts with an instructor in order to determine the reason for failure. Accidental pregnancies were classified as biological failures, user failures, or undetermined failures. A biological failure was recorded when the couple had a good understanding of the method and, as far as could be determined, had carried out the instructions faithfully. User failure was recorded when the pregnancy resulted from errors by the couple that the instructor could determine and explain to them or when the couple had neglected to use the technique properly. Undetermined failure was recorded when insufficient information existed to permit the instructor to determine the reason for failure. The failure rate for each category was calculated using the Pearl formula:[33]

$$\frac{\text{Number of accidental pregnancies}}{\text{Number of cycles}} \times 1200 = \text{Failure rate per 100 women years}$$

It was assumed that 12 consecutive menstrual cycles were equivalent to one year of ovulation method use. Since the method can be used either to prevent or to achieve pregnancy, those couples attempting the latter were dealt with separately.

Study population. The ages of the 371 women ranged from 19 to 48 years, with a mean age of 28 years. Respondents averaged two children per couple. Of the 371 women, 200 (59 percent) had previously used artificial methods of birth control. Seventy-five percent of these had used an oral contraceptive. Thirty-five of the pill users had experienced one or more undesirable side effects. One woman has been hospitalized following a cerebral thrombosis, and another suffered pulmonary embolism attributed to oral contraceptive use. Additionally, four women in the study suffered thrombophlebitis of the lower extremities. Other undesirable side effects reported were severe headaches, depression, and the lack of sex drive. All these women reported that their private physician attributed these findings to taking the pill.

Results. Three hundred twenty-nine women, or 89 percent, used the ovulation method to prevent pregnancy. Of these 329 women, 92 percent were using the method successfully after one year. A total of 27 women (8 percent) became pregnant. Of these 27 pregnancies, 18 were attributed to user failures, 6 were considered undetermined failures, and 3 were thought to be biological failures. The overall failure rate of the 329 couples using both preovulatory and postovulatory phases of the menstrual cycle for coitus through 3,354 cycles was 9.6 pregnancies per 100 women years. The 9.6 pregnancies per 100 women years are attributed to 1.1 biological failures, 6.4 user failures, and 2.1 undetermined failures. Therefore, only 3.2 (1.1 + 2.1) pregnancies per 100 women years can be attributed to the ovulation method used to the best of a couple's ability. It is interesting to note that 75 percent of those in the group labeled "user failures" intended to use the ovulation method again after pregnancy.

Of the 42 women who used the ovulation method to achieve pregnancy, 14 (33 percent)

*The complete questionnaire is available from Sr. Leona on request.

conceived within 1 year. Ten of the 14 women had no previous pregnancies. Prior to using the ovulation method, 7 women had used the basal body temperature method for 3 to 7 years to determine if ovulation occurred. Three women had taken a fertility drug for at least 1 year without success. One woman who had been unsuccessful for 7 years in achieving pregnancy using the temperature method reported success utilizing the ovulation method.

Until the couple gained confidence in the method, voluntary follow-up counseling services were provided and recommended to determine the woman's understanding of applying the method. Seventy-five percent of the women who did not utilize follow-up sessions had used the rhythm method prior to learning the ovulation method and thus were more familiar with the mechanical aspects of the ovulation method. All 36 women who returned for 3 to 6 sessions had previously been on the pill, reported considerable mucus, and so needed more counseling.

One year after training, the respondents were asked various questions to ascertain major difficulties in using the method (see Table). Women who indicated difficulty in interpreting their own mucus patterns stated that they gained confidence with each month's experience. Seventy-three percent of the couples took 2 months, 22 percent took 3 months, and 5 percent took 4 to 6 months before they gained complete confidence in using the ovulation method.

TABLE: Number of Responses To Ascertain Difficulties with the Ovulation Method

	RESPONSES		
QUESTIONS	YES	NO	NO RESPONSES
Experienced difficulty in interpreting own symptoms	244	127	
Days of abstinence a hardship in marriage (too much)	53	318	
Feel confident in using the ovulation method	279	92	
Follow-up sessions were helpful	272	7	92*
Would recommend the ovulation method to others	308	20	43

*Had no sessions.

DISCUSSION OF THE STUDY

The study was designed to determine the effectiveness of the ovulation method using the preovulatory and postovulatory phases of the cycle as determined by the cervical mucus symptom as a means of avoiding conception as well as a means of achieving pregnancy where women were otherwise unsuccessful. The study was also designed to determine the degree of satisfaction in using this method of family planning. The unplanned pregnancy rate of 9.6 per 100 women years in this report of the ovulation method is lower than those given in the first reported prospective field trial in Tonga, which revealed 25 pregnancies per 100 women years,[34] and in the Australian study reported by Ball, which gave a pregnancy rate of 21 per 100 women years.[35]

A study using the ovulation method in combination with the basal body temperature method in London reported by Marshall also reveals a higher pregnancy rate of 22 per 100 women years.[36] Marshall had earlier reported another study that used only the basal body temperature method with one group of women using the postovulatory phase and another group using both the pre- and postovulatory phases. For the group who confined coitus to the postovulatory phase only a 6.6 pregnancy rate per 100 women years was reported, while the rate for the group who used both the pre- and postovulatory phases revealed a pregnancy rate of 19.3 per 100 women years.[37]

Again, when coitus is not limited to the postovulatory phase, the overall 9.6 pregnancy rate in the St. Vincent study is lower than these figures. No valid comparisons can be made between the ovulatory and the basal body temperature methods using the postovulatory phase because no research has been reported in this area.

The ovulation method of family planning is free of undesirable biological side effects as well as free of the use of chemical or mechanical means of contraception. Although this study of the ovulation method shows 9.6 pregnancies per 100 women years, it indicates a 3.2 pregnancy rate per 100 women years in couples who are highly motivated to prevent pregnancy. This figure is higher than that given for oral contraception, reported at 1.0. It compares favorably with the 3.4 rate reported for the intrauterine device, the 12.0 rate reported for the diaphragm, the 14.0 rate reported for the condom, 18.0 for coitus interruptus, 24.0 for the rhythm method, and 31.0 for the douche method.[38] And weighing risk/benefits, one may conclude that the ovulation method, with a 3.2 pregnancy rate without risk, weighs favorably versus the contraceptive pill.

As with all natural methods of family planning, the ovulation method requires a period of abstinence. Allowing couples to utilize the day(s) in the preovulatory as well as in the infertile postovulatory phases decreases the number of abstinence days. There are no reported studies relative to problems with the period of abstinence. Based on the questionnaire used in this study, 318 out of 371 (86 percent) respondents did not find the required abstinence too much or a hardship in marriage.

The ovulation method also helped the women who used it to become pregnant, since 33 percent succeeded after failing with the basal body temperature method or with fertility drugs.

Because of its lack of side effects and its high success rate, the ovulation method of family planning has proved to be a viable and effective alternative to technological means of birth control.

REFERENCES

1. E. B. Connell, "The Pill Revisited." *Family Planning Perspective*, vol. 7, no. 2, 1975, pp. 62–71.
2. W.H. Inman and M. P. Vessey. "Investigation of Deaths from Pulmonary, Coronary and Cerebral Thrombosis and Embolism in Women of Childbearing Age," *British Medical Journal*, vol. 2, 1968, pp. 193-199.
3. E. R. Brickerstaff, *Neurological Complications of Oral Contraceptives*. Clarendon Press, Oxford, England, 1975, pp. 94–95.
4. L. M. Hellman, "Safety of Oral Contraceptives," *Texas Reports on Biology and Medicine*, vol. 25, 1967, pp. 318–333.
5. F. G. Arthes, P. E. Sartwell, and E. F. Lewison, "The Pill, Estrogens and the Breast, Epidemiologic Aspects," *Cancer*, vol. 28, 1971, pp. 1391–1394.
6. H. B. Taylor, "Oral Contraceptives and Pathologic Changes in the Breast," *Cancer* vol. 28, 1971, pp. 1388–1390.
7. "Female Cancer Death Rates, by Site, United States, 1930–1969," *CA—A Cancer Journal for Clinicians*, vol. 24, 1974, p. 7.
8. *Oral Contraceptives and Health—An Interim Report from the Oral Contraceptive Study of the Royal College of General Practitioners*, Pitman, New York City, 1974.
9. H. R. Barber, E. A. Graber, and J. J. O'Rourke, *Are Pills Safe?* Thomas, Springfield, IL, 1969, pp. 24–31.
10. H. Gershberg, M. Hulse, and Z. Javier, "Hypertriglyceridemia During Treatment with Estrogen and Oral Contraceptives: An Alteration in Hepatic Function?" *Obstetrics and Gynecology*, vol. 31, 1968, p. 186.

11. J. K. Baum, J. J. Bookstein, F. Hoitz, and E. W. Klein, "Possible Association Between Benign Hepatomas and Oral Contraceptives," *The Lancet*, vol. 2, 1973, pp. 926–929.

12. D. L. Contostalros, "Benign Hepatomas and Oral Contraceptives," *The Lancet*, vol. 2, 1973, p. 1200.

13. "Liver Tumours and Steroid Hormones," editorial, *The Lancet*, vol. 2, 1973, p. 1481.

14. "Liver Tumours and the Pill," editorial, *British Medical Journal*, vol. 3, 1974, p. 3.

15. *Royal College of General Practitioners Study.*

16. Boston Collaborative Drug Surveillance Program, "Oral Contraceptives and Venous Thromboembolic Disease, Surgically Confirmed Gall Bladder Disease, and Breast Tumours." *The Lancet*, vol. 1, 1973, pp. 1399–1404.

17. E. P. Levy, A. Cohen, and F. C. Fraser, "Hormone Treatment During Pregnancy and Congenital Heart Defects," *The Lancet*, vol. 1, 1973, p. 611

18. A. H. Nora and J. J. Nora, "Birth Defects and Oral Contraceptives," *The Lancet*, vol. 1, 1973, pp. 941–942.

19. A. H. Nora and J. J. Nora, "A Syndrome of Multiple Congenital Anomalies Associated with Teratogenic Exposure," *Archives of Environmental Health*, vol. 30, 1974, p. 30.

20. D. T. Janerich, J. M. Piper, and D. M. Glebatis, Oral Contraceptives and Congenital Limb Reduction Defects *New England Journal of Medicine*, vol. 291, 1974, pp. 697–700.

21. J. T. Lanman and A. Jain, "Association of Oral Contraceptives and Congenital Limb Reduction Defects," The Population Council, office memorandum (mimeo), Oct. 4, 1974.

22. D. H. Carr, "Chromosomes after Oral Contraceptives," *The Lancet*, vol. 2, 1967, pp. 830–831.

23. S. Romcharon, F. Pellegrin, and E. J. Horg, *The Occurrence and Course of Hypertensive Disease in Users and Nonusers of Oral Contraceptive Drugs*, the Walnut Creek Contraceptive Drug Study: a prospective study of the side effects of oral contraceptives, vol. 2 ed. S. Romcharon, (DHEW Publication No. NIH 76–563), pp. 1–135.

24. W. T. Smith, *The Pathology and Treatment of Leucorrhea*, Churchill, London, 1855, cited by A. R. Abrabanel in "Artificial Reproduction of the Cyclic Changes in Cervical Mucus in Human Castrates," *Transactions of the American Society for the Study of Sterility*, 1946, pp. 46–62.

25. J. Sezuy and A. Vimeaux, "Contribution a l'etude des sterilites inexpliques"), *Gynecologie et Obstetrique*, vol. 27, 1933, pp. 346–358.

26. J. Sezuy and H. Simonmet, "Recherche de signes directs d'ovulation chez la femme" ("Research on Direct Signs of Ovulation in Women"), *Gynecologie et Obstetrique*, vol. 28, 1933, pp. 756–763.

27. C. G. Hartman, *Science and the Safe Period: A compendium of Human Reproduction*, Williams and Wilkins, Baltimore, 1962, p. 294.

28. B. B. Rubenstein, "The Relation of Cyclic Changes in Human Vaginal Smears to Body Temperature and BMR," *American Journal of Physiology*, vol. 119, 1937, pp. 635–641.

29. E. Viergiver and T. Pommerenke, "Measurement of the Cyclic Variations in the Quantity of Cervical Mucus and Its Correlation with Basal Temperature," *American Journal of Obstetrics and Gynecology*, vol. 48, 1944, pp. 321–328.

30. E. L. Billings, J. J. Billings, J. B. Brown, and H. G. Burger, "Symptoms and Hormonal Changes Accompanying Ovulation," *The Lancet*, vol. 1, 1972, pp. 282–284.

31. J. J. Billings, *The Ovulation Method*, Advocate Press, Melbourne, 1970.

32. J. J. Billings, *Natural Family Planning: The Ovulation Method*, Liturgical Press, Collegeville, MN, 1973.

33. R. Pearl, "Contraception and Fertility in 2,000 Women," *Human Biology*, vol. 4, 1932, p. 363.

34. M. C. Weissmann, L. Foliaki, J. J. Billings, and E. L. Billings, "A Trial of the Ovulation Method of Family Planning in Tonga," *The Lancet*, vol. 2, 1972, pp. 813–816.

35. M. Ball, "A Prospective Field Trial of the 'Ovulation Method' of Avoiding Conception," *European Journal of Obstetrics, Gynecology, and Reproductive Biology*, vol. 6, no. 2, 1976, pp. 63–66, *Excerpta Medica*.

36. J. Marshall, "Cervical-Mucus and Basal-Body-Temperature Method of Regulating Births; Field Trial," *The Lancet*, vol. 2, 1976, pp. 282–283.

37. J. Marshall, "A Field Trial of Basal-Body-Temperature Method of Regulating Births," *The Lancet*, vol. 2, 1968, pp. 8–10.
38. S. Kamron, M. D. Maghissi, and T. N. Evans, *Regulation of Human Fertility*, Wayne State University Press, Detroit, 1976, p. 31.

Appendix 11
The Ovulation Method and PP

By Marsha McKay

In June of 1977, I asked Planned Parenthood of Portland (Ore.) to sponsor me to teach the ovulation method of birth control in their own clinics. At the time, I was associated with an experimental college of the Oregon State University and a Naturopathic College Clinic, teaching the Ovulation, or "Billings," Method out of my own home. I was having a good success rate with the method, and wanted work with it in a clinic setting, where I would have the chance also to train others. Planned Parenthood was interested, a CETA (Comprehensive Education and Training Act) grant was applied for and secured . . . and one of Planned Parenthood's first formal courses in the Ovulation Method was off and running.

Now, just over nine months later, we have seen more than 350 clients; have seen some encouraging preliminary figures on contraceptive success; have won support and encouragement of others on the clinic staff; and have received both a highly favorable community reaction and wide interest from individuals learning more about the method. In this brief article, I want to tell readers of *PP News* a little about the program, how it works, and what factors they will want to bear in mind before considering a similar program for their own communities.

HOW THE METHOD WORKS

First, a reminder on what the Ovulation Method is. It is in the family of "periodic abstinence" methods—that is, methods of birth control which work not by drugs or devices, but by arranging the timing of sexual intercourse to occur during the least fertile period in a woman's monthly cycle. But unlike other, more traditional methods of this kind, the Ovulation Method does not involve either calendar calculations or basal temperature readings. It is based instead upon the manner in which the "cervical mucus"—what most women recognize as their normal vaginal discharge—varies at different stages in the mentrual cycle. Characteristics of cervical mucus change noticeably with changes in the levels of estrogen and progesterone in the cycle, and this helps the woman to detect when she may be fertile and when she may not.

One thing that I think has been very important to my own success at teaching this method is the fact that I have been using it myself successfully for the past three years. More than most methods of contraception, this one is very difficult to teach effectively if one does not understand it through direct experience.

PROGRAM DESIGN

We started the program with myself as instructor, and one full-time assistant, with the title clerk-typist. We began with two full-time staff because we wanted to do extensive statistical record-keeping and analysis. Classes were scheduled once a week, on Mondays, with a limit of 12 women or couples per class (this was later raised to 16).

The instruction for a woman wishing to use the method for birth control is in two parts. At the initial 2½-hour session, she is provided with basic background information and a chart. Then she goes home and charts her cycle for at least one month, during which time it is recommended that she abstain from coitus. When she has a complete cycle entered on the chart, she comes back and has an individual follow-up interview. The purpose of this interview is to make sure she has an understandable pattern, that she is checking and charting her cycle correctly, that she would not be taking chances on fertile days and that she feels good about what she is doing.

I had suspected for some time that there would be a considerable demand for the classes once they were publicized and offered through a reputable agency like Planned Parenthood. Most people haven't heard of the Ovulation Method, but once they do hear of it, many are interested. Now, several months after the start of the classes, they are fully-booked more than a month in advance. In all, nearly 300 women and couples have passed through the program.

Early Reports Encouraging

Five months after the course began, we prepared a profile of the clients, and some interesting patterns emerged. By contrast with most populations on which there are reports in the Ovulation Method literature (most of whom are Catholic, and with average family size of four or more), our population has been 75 percent childless. Fifty-two percent are single and independent; 31 percent married; and 11 percent living together but unmarried. Four in five of the clients are between the ages of 21 and 30, with more towards the higher end of the range than the lower. Sixty percent have had some college, and 25 percent have graduated.

One of the most interesting findings of this review was the number of women and couples who had some previous experience with one or another birth control method before trying the Ovulation Method. Almost all clients (99 percent) have used at least one method of birth control before: 31 percent, one method; 33 percent, two methods; 21 percent, three methods; and 14 percent, four of five methods. Almost three-fourths (71 percent) have used the birth control pill, and more than half (54 percent), the diaphragm. Clearly, by the time some women get through the other birth control options and haven't found anything compatible with their own health and personal needs, they are ready to try periodic abstinence and the regular checking and charting of mucus.

Though it is too early to make any firm conclusions about the success of our course, the first returns are encouraging. Between January and September 1978, 292 women attended the basic education session. Of these, 170 have come back for the first follow-up session (usually, a month to six weeks following the initial session). And of these, 120 have come back for a *second* follow-up session—from one month to six weeks after the first follow-up. Of these 120, just three had experienced "failures" with the method by the second follow-up visit, and all three knew they were fertile at the time they had intercourse. There have been no "method" failures—that is, failures among women who followed the rules exactly—among the women who have been contacted to date.

Role of Male Emphasized

One feature of the Ovulation Method which appeals to some couples is the important role of the male partner. In our program, men are encouraged to come to classes with their partners, and many do. This provides them with an opportunity to ask questions in an informal, supportive atmosphere and involves them, many for the first-time, in decisions involving birth control.

Sometimes men come to the follow-up and then the focus usually changes to integrating use of the method into the relationship. Many men are very interested in being part of birth control decisions and this method provides the perfect opportunity for them. Sometimes partners will work out a deal where the woman is in charge of checking her mucus and the man is in charge of charting it. Not only does this promote cooperation, but it heads off possible errors due to sloppy charting.

One of the most rewarding aspects of this program for me has been the opportunity to train others to teach the technique. I myself was trained as an instructor by a woman who had a great deal of experience with the method and wrote the book which I use with my classes— *Cycles of Fertility: The Ovulation Method* (by Gillette and Guren, published by the Ovulation Method Teacher's Association, 4760 Aldrich Road, Bellingham, WA 98225).

COMMUNITY SUPPORT

Another rewarding aspect of the program for me has been the support it has received from others in the affiliate. Our medical director has been very helpful, referring women to me for classes and answering my questions regarding women's bodies and complications. The nurses and doctors' assistants refer to me when a woman indicates any interest in the Ovulation Method. Some of the clinic personnel have themselves attended the class and use the method themselves. Two in-house educational sessions have been given for clinic staff to explain what the method is and how it works, and most of them now have a basic idea of how the method works—though there *is* some controversy among our staff as to its effectiveness.

We have made some effort, within the limits of time available, to involve others in the community in the program. I have given introductory presentations to the staff of two county Family Planning clinics, who now refer women to me for classes. And I have gone twice with Education Department staff on their regular birth control presentation visit to a local community college. Several of the students signed up for the class as a result of that presentation. Most of the referrals for the classes now are from friends who have taken the class and enjoyed it.

The Ovulation Method certainly cannot answer every woman's birth control needs. With care and discipline, however, it offers a fairly effective method of avoiding pregnancy that involves no health risks, is free of charge (after the instructional class), and can involve men to whatever degree is comfortable. It seems appropriate at this time that Planned Parenthood clinics should be aware of the growing interest in this form of fertility awareness, and consider either expanding their own services to include instruction in the method, or handling the need for it through referral to other agencies.

MEDICAL NOTE

As part of informed consent and the decision making process associated with contraceptive choice, individuals need to be provided with information about the effectiveness of all methods. The most reliable data on use-effectiveness (pregnancy rates experienced by good, bad and indifferent users within one year of use) of the various periodic coital abstinence (PCA) methods found a pregnancy *rate of 19.1%* (Ref). To place this in perspective, from the same study the pregnancy rates with other methods are as follows:*

Pill	*2%*
IUD	*4.2%*
Condom	*10.1%*
Diaphragm	*13.1%*
Foam, Cream, Jelly,	
Suppositories	*14.9%*

However, the more consistently an individual uses a method, the higher will be his/her effectiveness rate.

It is also important that counselors advise a woman who is contemplating the use of a method generally recognized as less effective to explore how she would manage an unexpected pregnancy prior to making her contraceptive choice.

—Louise B. Tyrer
Vice President for Medical Affairs, PPFA

---

*Vaughn, B., Trussell, J., Menken, J., and Jones, E. F., "Contraceptive Failure Among Married Women in the United States, 1970-1973", Family Planning Perspectives, Volume 9, Number 6, November-December, 1977

Author and Subject Index